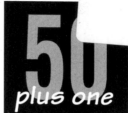

plus one

Medical Breakthroughs That May Help You Live Better

by
Michael Carney, Ph.D
&
Heather Z. Hutchins

ERIC DOBBY PUBLISHING

Eric Dobby Publishing Ltd
Random Acres
Slip Mill Lane
Hawkhurst
Cranbrook
Kent TN18 5AD
Email: publishing@gppbooks.com

ISBN 9781933766270

Printed by Berforts in the United Kingdom

Contents

Section 3: **The Human Factor**

Section 8: Follow Up Care

Section 9: Palliative Care

Section One:

Diagnostics

New Technology in Scanning

The Challenge

Only slightly over 100 years ago, the only way a physician could inspect the interior of the human body was to literally open up the body, look for symptoms or the types of conditions they suspected, note their findings—without any backup records besides perhaps a drawing—and close up the incision. The diagnosis made would then be based on the observations of the physician and the best memory of what he had seen. There was just as much danger in using this type of diagnostic technique as there was in operating and, often, a physician would simply perform an operation at the same time the examination was being done. Then came the miracle of x-ray technology which allowed a physician to view various areas of the body with radioactive waves. These x-rays would illuminate the interior of the body and the physician could look at the results during real time on a fluoroscope or by taking x-ray photographs and examining the results. X-rays were limited, however, in what they could show and overuse of the radiation could have serious side effects on the patient. Over the latter part of the 20th century physicians were able to begin using other forms of scanning that could accurately look at the interior of the body without the harm of x-rays, although x-rays are still being used. These new types of scans opened up whole new areas of diagnostic medicine. The technology is still being expanded and improved upon. The challenge is to know what the benefits or possible side effects of various scanning techniques might be, when the type of scan being proposed is appropriate to detection of a condition and what the physician is hoping to see from the scan. With the right knowledge, you can gain a better understanding of what scanning can do and where it is progressing in diagnosing medical conditions.

The Facts

Nuclear medicine has been a catch phrase for new scanning techniques, although, except for x-rays most modern scanners do not use radiation to look inside the body. Instead modern scanners use two different types of scanning techniques:

- Scanning a patient's body after the patient has ingested a radioactive substance, either a pellet or liquid that can be expelled from the body before it causes any harm, this is also used as an injection and

- scanning without the use of a tracer by placing the body in a scanning machine or running a portable scanning device over the area being examined.

Besides scanning, physicians can use other methods of examination that do not involve the opening of the body. These types of scans use miniature cameras for imaging and, in some cases, can take a sample of suspect tissue for later analysis. Some can even do some healing of the affected area as part of the scan.

- Angiograms use cameras on cables to explore the major arteries and the heart;
- Arthroscopes can look inside joints or soft tissue surrounding joints for evidence of disease or damage;
- Endoscopes are inserted into the gastrointestinal system through the esophagus and use a tube with a camera to look for potentially harmful conditions and
- Colonoscopes can explore the intestines and some surrounding organs by using a camera on a wire that is inserted into the body through the rectum,

Advent of magnetic resonance imaging revolutionized scanning, however, most scanning technology since its advances in the late 20th century produced only 2D images of the body. These were useful and less invasive, but not as accurate as possible. Now many scans can be made of an entire area of the body and combined by the computer to create a 3D model which can be manipulated by the radiologist or attending physician. 3D imaging can even be used during complex surgery.

The Solutions

The physician who will supervise your scanning and interpret the results is called a radiologist. The radiologist is a vital part of your medical team and will communicate with your primary care physician or specialist on your condition and recommend any follow-up tests. Often, the radiologist will examine the results of the scan via computer and be able to make a diagnosis very quickly.

Various scanning or medical imaging is used in various clinical contexts. Medical imaging is a sub-discipline of biomedical engineering, medical physics or medicine from research and development to image as well as modeling in biomedical engineering and research into new areas and techniques. Some of the most common types of medical imaging being currently used and improved are:

Ultrasonography or ultrasound scanning that uses pressure waves and echoes inside the tissue;

- Projection radiography which uses a probe with x-ray radiation that is absorbed at different rates in different types of tissues;
- Fluoroscopy which produces real-time images of the body interior in a similar way to radiography but uses a constant flow of x-rays and contrast media such as barium, iodine or air;

- Magnetic resonance imaging, MRI, which uses powerful magnets to polarize and excite hydrogen nuclei in water, producing a detectable signal which can be translated into images;
- Nuclear medicine uses images from gamma cameras to detect regions of biological activity associated with disease;
- Positron emission tomography, PET, used to detect disease of the brain and heart and uses a short lived isotope;
- Tomography which images a single plane of the body interior; this type of imaging is divided among linear tomography which moves an x-ray tube above the patient; poly tomography which has been largely replaced by computed tomography; zonography a form of linear tomography; orthopantomography, or OPT, which uses a complex movement to allow examination of the mandible; and\
- Computed tomography, CAT or CT which produces a 2D image of the structures in a thin section of the body and uses x-rays with greater ionizing radiation per dose.

One of the most interesting and potentially beneficial forms of new scanning is being researched right now. It is called electron spin resonance and could lead to a dramatic improvement in diagnosing serious illnesses such as heart disease, stroke, diabetes, septic shock and cancer. It is hoped this type of improved scanning will be able to provide a three-dimensional snapshot image of the chemical state of an organ such as the heart or lungs. Present scanning instruments do not have the sensitivity or speed to do this, but new measurement techniques and data analysis could possibly improve the sensitivity of the scan by 100 times or more. Electron spin resonance imaging instruments work in a similar way to MRI scans. Where MRIs use the magnetic properties of the protons in water to generate an image, electron spin resonance uses the magnetic properties of the electrons. This helps scan for chemical processes.

Improvements continue to be made in scanning techniques. Modern scanning techniques have benefited from wider dynamic range and reduction in over-and-under exposure to radiation. Other improvements have resulted in much faster imaging with a higher resolution. Companies such as Agfa, Eastman Kodak, Arraid, Edge, General Electric, Altaire, Integris, Toshiba and others are competing strongly for a share of the new market in medical imaging technology. Information about the latest scanning products from all of these companies is easily available online and you can ask your physician about what is available and what the benefits of each type of scan might be.

To save money on diagnosis and to improve the responses to a potentially harmful medical condition, physicians are following the Scan All Patients immediately method without scheduling a later appointment. This method will be especially used in a clinic, hospital or outpatient diagnostic center.

The Resources

Visit the following Websites for more information on new medical scanning technology:

Medical News Today, *www.medicalnewstoday.com*

Science Daily, *www.sciencedaily.com*

Advanced Imaging Magazine, *www.advancedimagingpro.com*

Medical Imaging, *www.medicalimaging.org*

Imaging Centers, *www.imaging-centers.com*

Radiology Journal, *www.radiologyjournal.com*

Medical Imaging News, *www.medicalimagingnews.com*

Several books can be very helpful in learning about medical scanning technology such as:

Harvard Medical School Family Health Guide (Free Press, 2004)

Progress in Medical Radioisotope Scanning (Oak Ridge Institute of Nuclear Medicine, 1962)

Current Medical Diagnosis & Treatment, 2006 (McGraw-Hill Medical, 2005)

Naked to the Bone: Medical Imaging in the Twentieth Century (Perseus Books Groups, 1998)

Functional MRI (Springer, 2000)

Cardiac CT Imaging: Diagnosis of Cardiovascular Disease (Springer, 2006)

DNA Testing

The Challenge

DNA provides the basic building blocks for the body. DNA governs everything from the color of your eyes to the density of your bones. Since its discovery in the 1950s, DNA has fascinated researchers who see it as not only a diagnostic tool, but also as a way to fight disease and genetic conditions. DNA is also an important tool in determining paternity of a child and in identifying perpetrators of a crime. It has become an almost irrefutable gauge to body traits and relationships between humans. Lately, DNA has been used more and more to predict potential health conditions that may affect a human. While the DNA testing cannot provide a cure, and is not a guaranteed measure, its use, combined with standard diagnostic procedures, including an examination of lifestyle, can alert patients of conditions that can be dealt with in the future, keeping in mind the adage that forewarned is forearmed. The challenge is to know when DNA testing can be useful, weighing its diagnostic significance and acting on what the DNA testing is indicating regarding potential medical conditions.

The Facts

With just a few exceptions, each of our body's cells contain a complete sample of DNA. For example, red blood cells do not contain DNA whereas white blood cells do. DNA is also found in most other living things including plants, animals and even bacteria. A strand of DNA is made up of four tiny building blocks: referred to as A, T, G and C blocks. These are also referred to as bases. Bundles of DNA form chromosomes that make up the cells in the body.

The most common use of DNA for medical testing over the last several years is for identifying potential cancer. Unlike other forms of medical testing that identify existing conditions, DNA testing is designed to predict the likelihood that a certain medical condition may occur. There is no guarantee that this condition will actually arise, but, when done properly, DNA testing can alert a patient and the physician to be aware of the potential condition and to perform further testing on a regular basis. As DNA testing becomes more and more prevalent, it will start to be commonly used to test for other medical conditions besides cancer.

One of the challenges in implementing DNA testing for cancer, heart disease and other medical conditions is making physicians more and more aware of the potential benefits of this type of testing. While physicians are always interested in using the latest reliable technologies in diagnosing and treating their patients, many are either unaware or resistant to the possible use of DNA testing. A patient should bring up this possibility with the physician and get that physician's opinion on whether he or she would use DNA testing and, if not, why this technology would not be employed.

To do testing of deceased family members to help determine a patient's predisposition to a possible medical condition, it is not necessary to dig up a body and extract samples from the remains. Unlike other forms of blood, fluid or tissue samples, all of your family medical history is contained in your DNA.

DNA testing for medical conditions depends on various specific methods and the nature of DNA. DNA testing for medical conditions uses a section of the Y-chromosome called non-coding DNA because it does not recombine or have known uses other than to fill in spaces between the genes. Since this DNA does not mix and mutates very slowly, it is the most beneficial for use in the genealogical applications for medical testing. If mitochondrial DNA testing is used, it examines the region known as the Hypervariable Region (HVR). A full mitochondrial sequence test may reveal medical conditions but will need to be analyzed by a specialist in this area. All test results, like other medical testing is not information for public consumption, unlike DNA testing for criminal purposes, and is meant to be only known and used by you and your physician.

The Solutions

DNA, whether it is obtained from blood or from other body tissues, must be handled carefully Contamination can vastly effect the reliability of the results of DNA testing. Avoiding contamination means researchers must keep equipment scrupulously clean and to properly store and segregate samples. Since contamination of a DNA sample is relatively easy, researchers must be careful not to overstate the infallibility of a DNA test and a physician must communication that with the patient.

DNA testing is not the only predictor of a patient's potential to acquire a serious medical condition and should not be relied upon as the only indicator. Besides DNA testing, a patient and physician should examine other factors that may enter into a patient developing cancer or a heart condition.

- A patient's family medical history, especially the history of any close relatives such as parents, grandparents, uncles and aunts and siblings;
- a patient's medical history showing prior development of certain medical conditions;
- lifestyle factors such as weight, diet, smoking, and use of alcohol or drugs and
- environmental factors such as exposure to toxins, lead based paint, particulates and asbestos containing materials.

One of the more promising areas DNA testing is being used for is to detect pote.......
heart conditions, especially when combined with a lengthy examination of a patient's
family history of heart disease. The test for this DNA is relatively simple and requires a
draw of blood. DNA testing of blood samples for heart conditions has been developed
primarily since 2004 and has shown a 90 percent penetration. This means that out
of 100 patients with a gene for a cardiovascular disease, 90 will actually develop the
disease.

Genetic testing will not determine the potential for every type of potential heart disease.
In its current state of development, genetic testing is most reliable for predicting
possible problems with arrhythmia, an irregular heart rate, coronary heart disease,
cardiomyopathy where the heart muscle becomes inflamed, congenital heart disease
and aneurysms.

Before discussing the possibility of using DNA testing to predict a potential disease,
you should be aware of the real advantages DNA testing as opposed to standard blood
testing.

- Complete blood group testing can allow discrimination of one person in several
  thousand. DNA testing can routinely provide exclusion probability in one in
  billions.
- Small sample sizes can be adequate in providing reliable results in DNA testing.
  If it is impractical to use blood for testing, DNA can be extracted from other body
  tissues even including hair follicles.
- DNA sampling is much more stable in comparison to the proteins found in blood
  samples. DNA is much more resistant to degradation by common environmental
  factors. DNA is much more long-lived that with the proteins found in other blood
  testing. Reliable information can be obtained from DNA samples that are many
  years old.

Although most DNA testing is done from blood samples, DNA testing companies
can utilize saliva/buccal cell sampling via simple swabbing and other non-invasive
collection techniques. A blood test may not be absolutely needed.

A growing trend in DNA medical testing is to use direct-to-consumer DNA testing.
This type of testing eliminates the need to go through a physician and uses a swab to
obtain and send DNA to a commercial testing house. While this type of testing adds
another layer of confidentiality. This is definitely a buyer-beware type of process, since
government regulators have no authority over these types of testing houses. Patients
can be prescreened to see if this testing is appropriate. The risk is that results can be
misinterpreted if they are analyzed by an improperly trained technician. For example
in detecting breast cancer through DNA testing, a woman may be told she is unlikely to
develop it based on the most common testing standards but may develop the disease
because the testing house did not properly analyze the sample for less common DNA
factors.

The Resources

Visit the following Websites for more information on DNA testing for medical conditions:

Scientific Testimony, *www.scientifc.org*

Ohio State University Medical Center, *www.osu.edu*

Colorado State University, *www.vivo.colostate.edu*

International Society of Genetic Genealogy, *www.isogg.org*

Boston News, *www.boston.com*

DNA Center, *www.dnacenter.com*

Several books can be very helpful in explaining DNA testing for medical conditions such as:

The Secrets of Medical Decision Making: How to Avoid Becoming a Victim of the Health Care Machine (Loving Healing Press, 2005)

Does It Run in the Family?: A Consumer's Guide to DNA Testing for Genetic Disorders (Rutgers University Press, 1997)

American Medical Association Family Medical Guide, 4th Edition (Wiley, 2004)

The Genetic Basis of Common Diseases (Oxford University Press, 2002)

American Medical Association Guide to Talking to Your Doctor (Wiley, 2001)

The Johns Hopkins Consumer Guide to Medical Tests: What You Can Expect, How You Should Prepare, What Your Results Mean (Rebus, 2001)

Dealing With Common Children's Conditions

The Challenge

Children can get sick just as often as adults and senior citizens. In some cases, children's diseases are specific for children of a certain age and can include infectious conditions, injuries, genetic illnesses and illness based on birth defects. Whatever the nature of the disease, diagnosing and dealing with children's diseases can present unique challenges that are not encountered for adults. Children can suffer equally from disease and the discomfort of dealing with a medical condition as a child can have a vast impact on the entire family. The challenge is to recognize what are the most common forms of children's diseases, what are the most effective ways to diagnose the disease, what treatment options are available and how they will impact the child in a negative way and what parents have to do at home to help identify and treat common children's medical conditions. Luckily, modern medicine and pediatrics, the study of children's diseases, is pointing out procedures in diagnosing and treatment that benefit both the child and the parent.

The Facts

The specialist dealing with children's medical conditions is called a pediatrician and deals almost exclusively with the treatment of children and the counseling to the entire family. Within the broad framework of pediatricians are specialists who play roles similar to that they do with adults. These specialties include internal medicine, orthopedic issues, neural conditions, treatment of injuries and others. You may be recommended to a pediatric specialist from your general pediatrician or family doctor or you may choose, based on your knowledge to send your child to a specialist.

Unlike adults, children may not understand what is being done to them in terms of diagnostic and treatment procedures and may very well act in a negative fashion when having to cope with medical procedures. This could include crying and overall resistance to the procedure being done to them because of its discomfort. Parents must find a pediatrician or family physician who is skilled in dealing with the psychological aspects of treatment and help the child patient understand what is being done and why. Parents need to recognize what their children can deal with and what it might take to help them through the process of diagnosis and treatment.

Children are just as susceptible to psychological ailments as adults. In some cases, these psychological and neurological ailments are more prevalent and more destructive than they might be for adults. These conditions include Attention Deficit Disorder, dyslexia, Tourette's Syndrome and miscellaneous eating disorders such as anorexia, overeating and bulimia.

Many times children will develop the same types of illnesses as adults but showing different symptoms and degrees of discomfort. The most common types of illnesses affecting children are:

- Sleep apnea or related difficulty sleeping through the night;
- Adenoid disorders;
- Tonsil disorders;
- Whooping cough;
- Measles, usually highly contagious but treatable with vaccinations;
- Mumps;
- Chicken pox;
- Croup;
- Rubella, a virulent form of measles;
- Meningitis, a contagious spinal disease;
- Head lice;
- Diarrhea;
- Constipation;
- Urinary tract infections;
- Ear conditions and
- Mouth conditions.

One of the more common forms of psychological disorder, which can also affect adults, is bipolar disorder. This condition is characterized by periodic mania activity from the child that could be destructive to him or her. Bipolar disorder symptoms usually include inflated self-esteem or grandiosity, decreased need for sleep, pressured speech, flight of ideas or racing thoughts, distractibility, increased goal-directed activity or excessive involvement in activities with a potential for painful consequences. It can be hard to diagnose these symptoms in younger children. Conduct disorder in adolescents, similar to bipolar disorder in children, can be marked with motives that are more hurtful, vindictive and antisocial. The keys to treating bipolar disorders in children is the careful use of medications and therapy.

The Solutions

A child, especially a younger child may have trouble explaining what symptoms they are feeling except for the sensation of being sick. Parents must be careful in talking to their children and asking certain questions that may help them recognize whether the child is experiencing real symptoms that need the attention of a physician or are simply displaying symptoms of a mild condition that can be easily diagnosed and treated at home without the need of the physician. Some of the most common questions and home diagnostics include:

- Where does it hurt? Follow up by palpating, or a applying pressure to the area to see if it hurts constantly or only when pressed.
- Are you feeling sick to your stomach? Has the child vomited or is experiencing diarrhea?
- Do you feel like you are running a fever? Follow up by taking the child's temperature and be aware of any sustained body temperature that is significantly and continuously higher than 98.6 degrees Fahrenheit.
- Do you have a sore throat or having trouble swallowing without pain? Follow up by using a small flashlight to look down the throat and check for white inflamed tissue or white patches.
- Do your ears hurt or are you having trouble hearing?
- Do you have a rash, where is it located and is it causing chronic itching? Follow up by looking at the area that may have a rash and look for inflamed skin or skin with obvious bumps on the affected area.
- Are you getting headaches?
- Is your vision blurry or are there dark parts of where you are looking?

One of the best ways to deal with childhood illness is to treat it before it manifests. This means making sure your child receives a proper series of vaccinations starting with a main shot and using periodic booster shots to combat potential diseases. The most common forms of vaccination fight polio, tetanus, measles, chicken pox, mumps and other infectious diseases. Some of these vaccinations may depend on an individual evaluation of risk factors, such as whether your child is part of day care or rides a school bus.

To understand and identify potential childhood disorders as opposed to traits shown through the normal growth process, parents need to understand their child's changing and emerging growth and development. This development can undergo a series of growth changes from infancy to adolescence. This growth and development not only includes the effects of physical changes in a child, but also the some of the changes in emotions, personality, behavior, thinking and speech. To help a child through these changes, it is vital parents promote good health as common problems develop.

Preventing infectious diseases is one of the largest challenges in children's hearth care. This prevention includes:

- Proper hand washing techniques;
- depending on the disease, taking certain precautions;
- following the nationally-recommended schedule for childhood immunization treatments and
- making sure children are properly taking their medications.

One of the most difficult decisions a parent will have to make is deciding whether a child needs to go through the trauma of surgery and how to help him or her through the process. Most childhood surgeries are designed to deal with:

- Further exploration of the condition for diagnosis;
- taking a biopsy of a suspicious lump;
- removing diseased tissues or organs;
- correcting an obstruction;
- repositioning structures to the normal orientation;
- redirecting channels;
- transplanting tissues or whole organs;
- implanting medical or electronic devices and
- improving the child's physical appearance through cosmetic surgery.

Like surgical issues for adults, parents must help their children through certain steps in preparing for and undergoing surgery. This includes receiving the surgical diagnosis made after an examination and testing, preoperative management that begins when surgery is decided upon and lasts until the child goes through the surgery, interoperative care that lasts from the time your child enters the operating room to when he or she enters the recovery area and postoperative management which lasts from the recovery room until a follow-up clinical examination is performed.

The Resources

Visit the following Websites for more information children's medical conditions:

American Academy of Pediatrics, *www.aap.org*

Wrong Diagnosis, *www.wrongdiagnosis.com*

Psychiatric Times, *www.psychiatrictimes.com*

Children's Hospital of Philadelphia, *www.chop.edu*

Find Articles, *www.findarticles.com*

About Pediatrics, *www.pediatrics.about.com*

University of Rochester Medical Center, *www.urmc-rochester.edu*

Several books can be very helpful in learning about children's conditions such as:

Education of Children with Medical Conditions (David Fulton Publishers, 2004)

Supporting Children with Medical Conditions (David Fulton Publishers, 2004)

Counseling Children with Chronic Medical Conditions (British Psychological Society, 2002)

Medical Conditions in School Children: A Guide for Teachers (Hodder and Stoughton Educational Division, 1988)

Shelter from the Storm: Caring for a Child with a Life-Threatening Condition (De Capo, 2005)

Consent, Rights and Choices in Health Care for Children and Young People (Blackwell Publishing Limited, 2001)

Non-Invasive
Technologies

The Challenge

Often people with challenging medical conditions will delay visiting a physician, even a Primary Care Physician, because they are afraid of the perceived pain and discomfort of invasive diagnostic and treatment procedures. They may be operating from old or wrong information and are not taking advantage of the latest improvements in non-invasive medical technologies. These technologies can use imaging and therapies that are either non-invasive or minimally invasive for the patient. The challenge is to maintain a basic awareness of non-invasive technologies, effectively discussing them as alternatives to more traditional treatments with your Primary Care Physician and have a reasonable expectation of what these technologies can accomplish as opposed to more invasive procedures. If it appears the non-invasive procedure is a workable alternative to more traditional methods, you owe it to yourself to thoroughly explore the procedure, determine your physician's use of it and then put forth the effort to pursue the non-invasive technology. Keep in mind these type of procedures, like many medical procedures are changing constantly and you need to keep up with those changes.

The Facts

The term non-invasive pertains to both medical procedures and to physical conditions caused by disease.

- A non-invasive medical procedure is one that does not penetrate the body or break the skin or body cavity. It most cases that means a non-invasive procedure does not involve an incision into any part of the body or the removal of body tissue for further study.
- A non-invasive medical condition is one that does not cause abnormal tissue growth. This growth, such as a neoplasm or tumor does not spread into surrounding tissue, invading other parts of the body.

Non-invasive procedures are nothing new in medicine. Literally for centuries physicians have been using various types of non-invasive procedures to assess and treat a patient. Only lately with the advent of advanced electronics and radiological devices, has non-invasive techniques grown into the vital part of medicine they are today. These non-invasive techniques became more and more important since the end of the nineteenth century.

A form of new non-invasive technologies is to use these technologies, when possible, to replace existing invasive technology. One primary and recent example is the use of computer-based 3D reconstruction to create a virtual colonoscopy, replacing the traditional method of inserting a colonoscope into a patient.

When non-invasive procedures are shown to be inadequate for diagnosis and treatment, physicians are using minimally-invasive procedures. These include hypodermic injection using a thin-needled syringe, endoscopy to access the digestive tract, Percutaneous surgery, laparoscopic surgery, coronary catheterization, angioplasty, stereotactic surgery and a variety of other developing minimally-invasive techniques.

Although it has been used for over 100 years, there have been very few changes in x-ray technology, until now. Researchers at the Brookhaven Laboratory are using x-rays from a national synchrotron light source, NSLS, using a low-dose experimental technique to visualize any bone and soft tissue in a manner not possible with more traditional x-rays. This method is also called diffraction enhanced imaging, DEI and can provide all the information now retrieved by x-rays as well as additional information on soft tissues previously measurable by MRI or ultrasound. DEI delivers a sharper image than these methods.

The Solutions

The various, most traditional and pervasive forms of non-invasive techniques have been available for over 100 years. As new non-invasive techniques have become more popular and improvements have been made in traditional non-invasive techniques, these procedures are still being highly used for diagnosis and treatment. Some of the most common forms of traditional non-invasive evaluation techniques include:

- Pulse-taking, auscultation of heart sounds and lung sounds through a stethoscope;
- body temperature evaluation using a thermometer;
- respiratory examination through evaluation of patient breathing;
- peripheral vascular examination by evaluating the skin condition;
- oral examination for evaluation of the tongue, tonsils and other oral tissues;
- abdominal examination through touch;
- external percussion and palpation;
- blood pressure measurement using a sphygmomanometer;
- changes in body volumes using a plethysmograph;
- audiometry to evaluate hearing and
- eye examinations.

Since the end of the nineteenth century, traditional non-invasive methods of diagnosis and treatment have been augmented with non-invasive techniques involving the increased use of specialized equipment. The most highly-used of these are:

- Ultrasonography and echocardiography using ultrasound waves for body imaging;
- x-rays used for radiography, fluoroscopy and computed tomography;
- using external magnetic fields for a variety of magnetic imaging that eliminates the radiation a patient incurs from x-rays;
- magnetic resonance spectroscopy;
- gamma camera and other scintillographical methods such as Positron Emission Tomography, PET scans and Single-Photon Emission Tomography, SPECT, that uses radioactive tracers in the body;
- infrared body imaging;
- diffuse optical tomography;
- elastography where stiffness and strain images of soft tissues are used to detect and classify tumors;
- posturography used to evaluate postural control in an upright stance;
- optical coherence tomography;
- bioluminescence imaging;
- dermatoscopy and
- gene expression imaging.

Besides new non-invasive technologies for diagnosis, modern physicians now have a variety of resources to use in non-invasive treatment. These methods of treatment eliminate much physical discomfort for a patient and include:

- Radiation therapy and radiosurgery which uses external atomic particles, such as protons, neutrons, photons and alpha particles, or gamma rays to destroy dangerous pathological tissues in the body;
- lithotripsy, a procedure that uses ultrasound shock waves to break down harmful urinary calculus;
- defibrillation to block heart fibrillation, an erratic heart beat, and restore normal heart rhythm;
- mechanical ventilation, such as an iron lung;
- transdermal patches which can deliver drugs when directly applied to the skin rather than relying on intravenous injections;
- biofeedback;
- Continuous Positive Airway Pressure, CPAP used to treat sleep apnea, a harmful interruption of normal breathing during sleep;
- Photodynamic therapy;
- therapeutic ultrasound;
- extracorporeal thermal ablation to heat diseased body tissues;
- photo-infrared pulsed bio-modulation and
- transcranial magnetic stimulation.

One of the most important aspects of non-invasive technologies involves the treatment of children or pediatric medicine. Children are less able to intellectually deal with the procedures being performed on them and are more likely to show distress. This is called Observed Behavioral Distress, OBD. To help ease this distress, physicians are using advanced cognitive behavioral therapy including filmed modeling, breathing exercises, imagery/distraction, positive incentives and behavioral rehearsal that significantly reduce OBD, heart rate and pain ratings among children.

Evaluating liver and kidney disorders has often involved uncomfortable invasive procedures such as endoscopy, where a camera is physically inserted into a partially-sedated patient. New tests, according to the latest research can detect liver and kidney diseases before symptoms are apparent and provide a faster way of evaluating a patient's response to disease treatment. This could mean eliminating a patient's need for costly and uncomfortable dialysis procedures. The new tests could virtually eliminate the need to take tissue biopsies. They can accurately measure response to uncomfortable drug treatments and allow clinicians to adapt their treatments to individual patient requirements. The tests work by identifying the amount of a cylokine molecule called monocycle chemoatrractant protein-1, MCP-1, that is found in the urine. MCP-1 is produced as a response to inflammation and can attract while blood cells to the affected areas. Overreaction of these white blood cells can cause vasculitis and organ damage. The test is relatively inexpensive, compared to dialysis, and very easy to take.

The Resources

Visit the following Websites for more information on non-invasive medical techniques:

Brookhaven National Laboratory, *www.bnl.gov*

University of California at San Diego, *www.health.ucsd.edu*

Journal of Pediatric Psychology, *www.jpeopsy.oxfordjurnals.org*

News-Medical, *www.news-medical.net*

Azonano, *www.azonano.com*

Medical News Today, *www.medicalnewstoday.com*

Several books can be very helpful in explaining non-invasive medical techniques such as:

Medical Imaging Techniques: A Comparison (Plenum Pub, 1979)

Healing Hands: Simple and Practical Reflexology, Techniques for Developing Good Health and Inner Peace (O Boos, 2005)

Medical Image Computing and Computer-Assisted Intervention (Springer, 2004)

Statistical Analysis of Medical Data: New Developments (Hodder Arnold Publication, 1998)

Harvard Medical School Family Health Guide (Free Press, 2004)

Advances in Healthcare Technology: Shaping the Future of Medical Care (Springer, 2006))

5

Investigating the Possible Benefits of Stem Cell Research

The Challenge

The issue of researching and using stem cells has been controversial and the subject of legislation and political campaigns for many years. Stem cells use living cells to provide treatment for a variety of chronic illnesses that are untreatable through traditional methods. The benefits are quickly pointed out by advocates of using stem cells. Opponents, who view embryonic stem cell research as an improper use of unborn fetuses, say there is no real evidence that stem cell treatments will work and is not worth the risks and moral compromise. You should know what is currently available in stem cell research, what its possible implications to the treatment of disease are and where this research is leading.

The Facts

Stem cells are different from regular or undifferentiated cells in many ways. Researchers believe stem cells can be grown into almost any kind of cell and be used to replace damaged cells, especially neural cells.

Despite opposition, stem cell research is one of the fastest growing aspects currently being pursued in medical research. Experts believe literally billions of dollars are being poured into the research, but most of this funding is from private resources and not the government.

Although stem cells taken from embryos is the most known and controversial use of stem cells, there are several sources for acquiring stem cells.

- Embryonic cells from unborn fetuses;
- adult cells extracted from bone marrow (the richest source) or from the peripheral system and
- spinal cord cells.

Like blood types, there are a number of common stem cells, however, the usefulness of these cells diminishes when they are not used on a family member. Scientists are developing methods of increasing transferability and reduce possible risk.

Embryonic cells are the most controversial in acquiring stem cells. The cells are removed from a fetus before the embryo cells begin to differentiate. At this time an embryo is referred to as a blastocyst. Each blastocyst contains about 100 stem cells which can be kept alive indefinitely and grown in cultures, where the stem cells double in number every two to three days. A replicating set of stem cells is called a stem cell line because all the material comes from the same fertilized human egg. In August, 2001, President Bush authorized the use of 15 existing stem cell lines with help from federal funding. Other stem cell lines are available for research, but this research is not funded by the government.

Some researchers claim they have used stem cells to produce several nerve growth factors. These nerve growth factors are actually proteins which stimulate the survival and regeneration of neurons, which help repair damaged nerve cells.

Beyond the ethical considerations there are very real practical differences between the use of adult and embryonic stem cells.

The advantages of adult stem cell research include:

- Bone marrow and umbilical stem cells seem to be as flexible as the embryonic cells.
- Recipients who receive their own stem cells will not reject them and not form tumors.
- Adult stem cells are relatively easy to acquire.
- No harm comes to the donor of adult stem cells.

The disadvantages of adult stem cell research include:

- They are sometimes difficult to obtain in large numbers.
- Adult stem cells may not live as long as embryonic stem cells.
- Adult stem cells are less flexible and may be harder to use to form other tissue types.

The advantages of embryonic stem cell research include:

- Embryonic stem cells appear to have the potential to form any type of cell.
- One embryonic stem cell line can possibly provide an endless source of cells with defined characteristics.
- Embryonic stem cells from in vitro fertilization are much more available.

The disadvantages of embryonic stem cell research include:

- Embryonic stem cells from a random donor are more likely to be rejected after transplantation.
- Embryonic stem cells may promote the growth of tumors or form new tumors.
- Some believe the use of embryonic stem cells results in the destruction of human life.

The Solutions

Because of stem cells supposed ability to grow into neural cells, researchers believe they can be used in the treatment of diseases that are now seen to be debilitating and incurable. These include Alzheimer's Disease, dementia and Parkinson's Disease. Having these diseases now usually means dealing with constantly-worsening symptoms, where stem cells might provide an actual cure.

Many researchers believe stem cells can be used to replace almost any dead cell. This can be especially helpful in replacing healthy cells killed by standard radiation or chemotherapies for a variety of cancers.

Extracting stem cells from bone marrow can be painful for the patient with the destruction of other cells part of the extraction process. Acquiring peripheral stem cells is less painful but also takes more time and this can be a factor when time is of the essence in treating a condition.

Another rich source of stem cells are from the umbilical cord. This can be especially useful if the family plans ahead. The cells can provide a perfect match when the family properly plans. Cord cells can be used by the mother and father or possibly other distant family members. The more removed the member, the less benefit the cells will have. The cord cells are extracted during pregnancy and stored in a cryogenic tank. These offer a type of insurance against future needs.

Those who oppose embryonic stem cell research say it kills human life because acquiring the cells means the destruction of an unborn embryo. Embryonic research advocates say the embryo has developed no human characteristics. They argue that new stem cell lines exist due to the often-used practice of in vitro fertilization. Advocates claim new human lives will not be created just for the purpose of experimentation. They also point out that many fertilized human eggs have already been banked but are not being made available for research.

There have been documented medical reasons arguing against the use of stem cells to treat disease. Almost 20 percent of mice treated for Parkinson's Disease have died from brain tumors. Embryonic stem cells stored over a long period of time have developed the chromosomal anomalies that can cause cancers. From a pragmatic view, it may be more worthwhile to pursue adult or umbilical stem cells rather than embryonic cells.

One of the more discussed aspects of stem cell research is the controversial proposal that women be paid to donate their eggs. The eggs could be used to impregnate infertile women or to provide stem cells. Opponents compare this practice to the odious idea of selling body parts.

Despite the arguments promoting some types of stem cell acquisition and research, there are currently federal laws that restrict access to embryonic stem cells, especially in the case of aborted fetuses. Proponents of these laws say they prevent the destruction of human lives. Researchers argue these laws needlessly restrict research into a potentially very beneficial type of medical treatment. Right now it appears unlikely that the federal government will allow experimentation with embryonic stem cells. Researchers must still rely on using adult or umbilical stem cells for research and treatment.

The Resources

Visit the following Websites for more information on stem cell research:

Stem Cell Research Facts, *www.stemcellreasearchfacts.com*

Life Issues, *www.lifeissues.net*

All About Popular Issues, *www.allaboutpopularissues.org*

National Institute of Health, *www.nih.gov*

Stem Cell Research, *www.stemcellresearch.org*

American Association for the Advancement of Science, *www.asas.org*

Several books can be very helpful in making you understand stem cell research such as:

Stem Cell Research: Medical Applications and Ethical Controversy (Checkmark Books, 2006)

The Stem Cell Divide: The Facts, the Fiction and the Fear Driving the Greatest Scientific, Political and Religious Debate of our Time (Lippincott, Williams and Wilkins, 1998)

Stem Cell Research: New Frontiers in Science and Ethics (University of Notre Dame Press, 2004)

Stem Cell Research: Issues and Bibliography (Novinka Books, 2006)

6

Understanding the Primary Care Physician Role

The Challenge

Almost all of your medical attention will start with your primary care physician. This type of doctor used to be called a general practitioner, but the name of primary care physician or PCP is actually much more descriptive. It accurately indicates that a PCP is the place to go to when you need to attend to a yearly examination or consult with regarding concerns over a medical condition that has taken you by surprise. You will establish a unique relationship with your PCP and find yourself relying on him or her to initially evaluate your overall health, advise you regarding lifestyle influences on your health and be the first to see you about your condition. There are some conditions whose treatment will begin and end with a visit to your PCP, others that will be referred to specialists depending on the perceived condition and what specialist might be the next logical step in dealing with the condition. Your PCP will help you monitor your condition after you have started treatment with other physicians and provide a vital link between you and your specialists. They can help you after your formal treatment by monitoring your condition and how the treatments are affecting it. They can offer worthwhile advice on what you need to do to further understand and deal with your unique condition. In most cases, your medical insurance will require you to start your medical treatment with your primary care physician before you start incurring the costs of visiting a specialist and undergoing more elaborate treatments. The challenge is to understand what a PCP can do for you, locating a PCP you feel comfortable with and evaluating their ongoing performance, including ability to communicate, to help you maintain a productive relationship. Finding a good PCP is essential to your medical care and you need to take the time to reliable advice on who to see as you work on maintaining your good health.

The Facts

Primary care physicians, in a sense, are medical specialists who generalize in diagnoses and treatments. Usually PCPs are trained in family practice, general practice, pediatrics and internal medicine. In some cases, medical insurance carriers, especially HMOs, will consider gynecologists as PCPs for the care of women and have allowed certain subspecialists to take on PCP responsibilities for selected patients including allergists and nephrologists. Sometimes PCPs may include nurse practitioners, physician assistants and naturopathic physicians.

Besides the usual aspects of a PCP examination that would include a visual inspection of the body and looking at other relatively simple indicators, such as examining the eyes, ears, throat and palpating to inspect the prostate gland. A PCP may also be able to evaluate the results of more complicated and involved medical tests. These might include interpreting the results of blood tests or other patient samples, electrocardiograms taken in the PCP's office or x-rays. More complicated tests are performed by a specialist, recommended by the PCP, who has increased experience and a practice that has a patient volume that renders a risky procedure safer for the patient.

The medical insurance carriers usually refer to PCPs as gatekeepers. This is because the PCP is considered the initial contact for most patients and help direct them to the needed specialists. The PCP acts on behalf of the patient to collaborate with referred specialists, coordinate care from a variety of sources and act as the primary repository for patient records. Continuous care for a patient by a PCP is especially useful when the patient has ongoing conditions such as diabetes and hypertension.

For a variety of reasons including the perception of increased income or ability to treat patients for specific conditions, PCPs are becoming in short supply in developed countries. According to the American Academy of Family Physicians, half of internal medical residents chose to be PCPs in 1998, but by 2006, over 80 percent became specialists. The median income of specialists in 2004 was twice that of PCPs and that gap is widening. Because of these factors, more and more PCPs in the United States are foreign-born physicians.

PCPs are sometimes referred to as family physicians. This means the PCP not works with one patient's symptoms and general health issues but also can work with an entire family. This not only makes receiving primary medical care easier for many families, but allows the PCP to evaluate the medical condition based on environmental and lifestyle factors of the entire family and living space.

The Solutions

Finding a good PCP can take some time and effort. Most communities will have a find-a-doctor service and this can be a good place to start looking. Some PCPs will offer online information including basic information on education, where he or she is located, a general idea of fees and co-payments for office visits and a list of any specialties over and above a PCP service. A friend or family member can help you find a good PCP and give you an idea of his or her experience. All of these are factors to use in making your initial selection, but you may decide to choose a different PCP once you have made your initial visit.

As you work on selecting a good PCP, you need to examine their set of skills and existing scope of practice. These are normally basic diagnosis of medical condition and non-surgical treatment of common illnesses and conditions. There are certain diagnostic techniques a PCP will use in their practice:

- Interviewing the patient to collect the current information on the patient's evident symptoms;
- taking and questioning prior medical history and other health details and
- doing a thorough physical examination.

A PCP is only as good as the information the patient supplies regarding the medical condition. The relationship must be seen as a partnership where the patient has to do the work to evaluate their symptoms and then adequately communicate them. This communication includes alerting the PCP to any changes in a medical condition, its progress and how it is responding to prescribed treatments.

The normal method of a PCP is to collect the essential data from the patient, either from the patient's detailed medical information for a physical examination and basic office tests. After collecting this data, a PCP will arrive at a differential diagnosis, and with the help of the patient, will arrive at a plan of further diagnoses or treatments. These may include specialist referral, medications, therapies, diet or changes in lifestyle, education and follow-up of treatments.

Medical care practitioners and medical insurance companies have recognized the shortage of PCPs and are taking actions in changing their models of care to return us to a time when PCPs were the core of medical care. These models stress trust in a PCP and how the PCP fees are more speedily and adequately paid by the medical insurance carrier. The trust issue is considered critical in using a PCP.

As you make your first visit to a potential PCP there are several questions you should be prepared to ask to evaluate the PCP and help determine the best way to work with him or her as a team in treating your medical conditions:

- What do I need to expect on a first visit? This visit should involve taking a thorough history and examination including basic tests of blood and urine samples.
- Does the PCP have a subspecialty? Is your PCP a general practitioner, internist or family practitioner. For example, an internist specializing in cardiology may be your best choice if you believe you are suffering from a heart condition.
- What are the PCPs hospital affiliations?
- What are the office's fees and billing systems?
- Who will cover the practice if the PCP is absent?
- Will the PCP do telephone consultation?
- Does the PCP make house calls. Some doctors still do this which can be especially helpful if you are a homebound handicapped person.

The Resources

Visit the following Websites for more information on the role of primary care physicians:

National Association for Children of Alcoholics, *www.nacoa.net*

The Health Pages, *www.thehealthpages.com*

Managed Care, *www.managedcaremag.com*

American Academy of Family Physicians, *www1.aafp.org*

National Library of Medicine, *www.ncbi.nlm.nih.gov*

Institute of Medicine, *www.iom.edu*

American College of Physicians, *www.acponline.org*

Several books can be very helpful in learning about the role of primary care physicians such as:

Procedures for Primary Care Physicians (Mosby, 2003)

Communication in Medical Care: Interaction Between Primary Care Physicians and Patients (Cambridge University Press, 2006)

Cardiology for the Primary Care Physician (Current Medicine Group, 2005)

Behavioral Medicine in Primary Care (McGraw-Hill Medical, 2003)

Treatment Guidelines for Medicine and Primary Care, 2006 (Current Clinical Strategies, 2006)

Psychiatry for Primary Care Physicians (American Medicine Association Press, 2003)

7

Knowing What Questions to Ask Your Primary Care Physician or Specialist

The Challenge

Communication with your primary care physician, specialist or other caregivers is essential to your healthcare. This communication depends on how good the physician is in telling you what is going on with your medical condition, avoiding the overuse of confusing medical jargon you may not easily understand and taking the time to properly communicate with you during an examination or visit. However, you cannot just rely on your physician to supply the information you need to assess and make decisions on your condition. You must also be willing to ask questions of your physician and use the answers to create follow-up questions. Asking these questions will not only help you better understand the nature of your condition, but will help you establish a good working relationship with your physician. The challenge is to feel comfortable in taking the time to ask your physician questions you need answered, being able to do your research ahead of time to ask the proper questions and avoid wasting your and your physician's time and then following up on the answers you receive. Asking questions may make you mildly uncomfortable, but a good physician will expect you to do this and should welcome the opportunity to educate you and your family on your condition and what can be done about it.

The Facts

Many people believe that asking questions indicate you are ignorant or do not have the ability to process the information. They fear what they think is a dumb question. But, the old adage is true. The only dumb questions are the ones we do not ask. Your physician or caregiver should not give off a judgmental attitude regarding your condition and encourage you to ask anything that concerns you regarding your health.

There are two basic times you should be asking questions of your doctor. One is prior to your visit and the others are part of your business. Before you visit a new doctor you should find out how large the staff is, how long the physician has been practicing, is the physician covered by your medical insurance, what is the policy on delays in an examination or treatment and what the physician normally charges and whether they will accept debit or credit cards.

A visit to your physician, whether primary care physician, should not leave you feeling confused about what you have been told. You should believe that your questions have been properly answered. If you think of things you should have asked your physician, but neglected to, or realize you need to clarify some information, contact the physician either by the phone or via email. Your physician or his or her nurse should get back to you as soon as possible. You may want to take family members or friends into the consultation and conclusion portions of the physician visit to make sure you have asked the questions you need to know and help you remember the answers. Take a pad of paper with your questions written on it and mark down the answers you hear for later review.

The Solutions

Asking questions goes both ways. Certainly you may want to ask your physician something you have been told, but you must expect your physician is going to ask you questions that are not included in a standard new-patient form. These questions might be generated from what your primary care physician sees on an examination and must be answered honestly to allow your doctor to accurately diagnose and treat your condition. For example, many people do not tell the truth when asked questions about perceived bad habits. Some of the questions you should expect to hear are:

- Are you having any shortness of breath?
- Are you experiencing any pain?
- When was the last time you visited a physician?
- Do you have any allergies to medications, especially antibiotics?
- Are you experiencing any trouble sleeping? Do you know if you snore loudly or your breathing stops while you are asleep?
- Are you having constant nausea?
- Are you experiencing any sexual dysfunction including erectile disorder?
- Are your flows constant during your menstrual cycle?
- Are you having trouble starting a bowel movement or urinating or are you experiencing diarrhea and a constant urge to urinate?
- Do you use tobacco products such as cigarettes, cigars or pipes? Are you using smokeless tobacco including snuff and chewing tobacco? How much do you smoke per day?
- Do you drink alcoholic? How many alcoholic drinks do you take a day?
- Do you use other drugs such as marijuana, cocaine, heroin, hallucinogens and methamphetamines?

Understanding your physician's responses to your important questions is essential to good conclusion for medical purposes. Keep these suggestions in mind as you work on understanding what your doctor is telling you:

- Be sure to ask all the questions you need to if you feel you cannot understand what you are being told.

- Instead of paper notes you can bring in a tape recorder to record the conversation to help you assist in your recollections of the discussion.
- Your doctor can also write down what you have been told, relying on having office staff transcribing any recorded notes and sending them to you.
- Ask your doctor if there is any printed material or appropriate online resources that can help you better understand your condition.
- Request a referral to another source or professional organization for where you can go for more information.
- Make sure you talk just as much to nurses, technicians, therapists and pharmacists just as much as you would to your physician. They can provide just as valuable information as the physician.

Be prepared to answer questions regarding your family history. Your primary care physician will be especially interested if there is any family history of heart disease, cancer and diabetes. These can be genetic ailments and, if your close relatives have had one of them, you may have an increased risk of disease. This is especially true of heart disorders. Expect to be asked questions about your family and do some research to find out what your immediate family might have had. Do not hold this information back for any reason from your physician.

Although your questions may depend on the specifics of your condition and medical history there are certain questions that should be asked almost every type of physician in diagnosing and treating your condition.

- What is the diagnosis?
- What might have caused the condition?
- Is this condition treatable?
- Should I be watching for any particular symptoms and when should I notify you if they occur?
- Would lifestyle changes affect my condition?
- How can my condition be treated?
- When will the treatment begin and how long will it last?
- What risks and side effects should I expect from this treatment?
- Are there any foods, drugs or activities I should avoid?
- What should I do if I miss any dose of medication?
- What other choices in treatment might I have?
- What type of tests will you prescribe?
- What will any tests show?
- How long will it take to get the results of my tests?
- Do I have to do anything special to prepare for the test?
- Do the tests have any significant side effects or risks?
- Will I possibly need additional tests later?

The Resources

Visit the following Websites for more information on asking the right questions of your physician:

Ohio State University, *www.medicalcenter.osu.edu*

National Eye Institute, *www.nei.gov*

National Institute for Health, *www.nih.gov*

Baptist Online, *www.baptistonline.org*

TTS Foundation, *www.ttsfoundation.org*

Dr. Donnica, *www.drdonnica.com*

Doctors Online, *www.geocities.com*

Several books can be very helpful in learning about asking the right questions of your physician such as:

What Your Doctor Hasn't Told You and the Health Store Clerk Doesn't Know: The Truth About Alternative Treatments and What Works (Avery, 2006)

Your Body, Your Health: How to Ask Questions, Find Answers, and Work With Your Doctor (Prometheus Books, 2002)

50 Plus One Questions to Ask Your Doctor (Encouragement Press, 2006)

How Long Will I Live?: And 434 Other Questions Your Doctor Doesn't Have Time to Answer and You Can't Afford to Ask (McMillan, 1976)

What Your Doctor Won't (Or Can't) Tell You: The Failures of American Medicine— And How to Avoid Becoming a Statistic (Berkley Trade, 2005)

How to Talk to Your Doctor: The Questions to Ask (Simon and Schuster, 1986)

8

Evaluating the Communication Process

The Challenge

A vital part of healthcare is communicating with your physicians. This means taking the time to ask questions and demanding your physicians take an equal amount of time to reply to these questions. More often than not, an important part of a good bedside manner for a physician is being willing to sit with a patient and discuss, in layman's terms, the patient's conditions. If a physician is unwilling to do this in a proper manner, and seems more interested in dashing off to the next appointment, this may not be a good fit for you. The challenge is to understand the nature of your possible condition, ask questions while the physician is examining you and demand you get the answers you need. Understanding and evaluating the communication process with your physicians and medical technicians is vital, but many people give this short shrift. You must put as much time into communicating as you would with any other aspect of your health care.

The Facts

Communication with a physician goes beyond discussion over medical procedures and can include business information. This information may be about insurance coverage, what insurance plans the physician participates in, how you will be billed and what provision a physician would have for phased billing. Make sure the office staff also is clear in their communication when they check you in and know who you should talk to if there is any dispute over a bill or explanation of procedures. A good support staff is just as important in communication issues as the physician is.

You and your physician are a team, probably the most important team you will ever be part of in your life. If you have any experience or knowledge of team sports you should understand the importance of clear communication in the success of your team. It is no different than with your medical team which may include your primary care physician, nurses and nurse practitioners, specialists, technicians or therapists. Good communication should address current problems as well as look ahead to other possible medical conditions. Many times physicians are juggling several elements in their practices, but once a physician is alone with you in an examination room, you are establishing a sacred bond with the physician. This will help allow you to get the attention you need and deserve from your physician.

Take the time necessary to note what diplomas or professional certifications your physician may have obtained. Be sure to ask questions about a physician's background. A good physician should have no problem in telling you why he or she is good at her practice and what can be offered to you.

The patient-physician communication encounter incorporates two important dimensions. Those are the instrumental and expressive dimensions. The instrumental element involves the physician's competence in performing the technical aspects of care such as the physical examination and prescription of treatments. The expressive element reflects the art of medicine including patient-perceived physician warmth and empathy and how the physician interacts with the patient.

The Solutions

Foreknowledge of your medical condition is vital to knowing how to communicate with your doctor. You can find more information about your medical conditions by picking up medical encyclopedias either from a book vendor or at the library. You can also visit medical informational Websites such as *www.webmd.com* to learn more about your medical condition.

Communicating with a physician is similar to communicating with any professional. You need to know what you must know and to take the time to get the information from your physician. Discourage your physician from using jargon and repeat the answers you are getting to make sure you are hearing the response properly. If you do not understand what is being told to you, do not feel too embarrassed to ask more questions or for a clarification. A good physician knows you are not a medical professional and should be willing to take the time and effort to help you understand what is being told to you.

Your responsibility as a patient in the communication process with your physician is to provide clear, concise and correct information regarding your history and medical symptoms. You should never lie about your behavior and you should believe your physician is not there to judge you, but to work with you to help in your health issues. Your physician's responsibility is to take the facts you provide and piece them together to provide discovery, diagnosis and a suggested plan of treatment. There are several things you can do to help with the communication process with your physician.

- Be as candid as you possibly can about your condition. Your physician needs to know exactly what type of symptoms you are experiencing.
- Do not waste your time or that of the physician's with extraneous information that has nothing to do with your current condition. Your family history is only important in how it might affect your symptoms and possible illness now.
- Prioritize your discussion with your physician by concentrating on just a few concerns to discuss during one visit.

- If you feel you need moral support or are in a situation of stress that may make it harder for you to properly communicate with your physician, you may want to consider bringing in a close family member or friend to your appointment and help you ask the right questions and understand what is being told you. A second set of ears can be very beneficial during a doctor appointment.
- Take written notes or ask your physician to provide you with printed material regarding your condition. Review the notes after the appointment and make sure you understand them and your needs have been properly answered. If you feel the communication was inadequate, call your physician or nurse for clarification.
- Repeat back what is being said to you and ask your physician to repeat vital information until you feel confident you are properly understanding it.
- Be organized when you visit a physician's office, especially during an initial visit, and come prepared with information about your symptoms, how long you have had them and what you have been doing on your own to deal with them. Be prepared to discuss your lifestyle and habits and be honest about them.
- Take along a comprehensive list of medications you are taking for other conditions including dosage and frequency. You may want to take in the actual medicine bottles.
- Take the time to feel comfortable you are exploring all of the treatment options for your condition. This will help you decide on an educated decision about your treatment plan.
- Follow through immediately and completely with the treatment plan. Do not improvise and change your treatment plan, based on its effects to your condition, without consulting your physician first. If your treatment is not working, do not just stay with it, but inform your doctor immediately.
- Make sure your physician tells you the best way to do any follow-up communication after the physical appointment. Depending on your comfort level, this may be email, phone calls or another visit in person.
- Be assertive during your physician visit in getting the answers you need, but avoid being aggressive. This perceived aggression can be misinterpreted and needlessly interfere with physician communication.

One of the most common methods in obtaining a physician, especially a primary care physician is to ask for a recommendation from family or friends. As part of getting this recommendation, be sure to ask the person giving the referral how they believe the communication process worked with the physician. You may be surprised at how little the person making the referral really understood the communication process and how the physician did not provide a good level of communication.

The Resources

Visit the following Websites for more information on physician-patient communication:

American Medical Association, *www.ama.org*

About Arthritis, *www.arthritis.about.com*

UK Patient Education, *www.mc.uky.edu/uk*

Ohio State University Medical Center, *www.medicalcenter.osu.edu/patientcare*

National Institute of Health, *www.nih.gov*

American Heart, *www.americanheart.org*

Several books can be very helpful in enhancing patient-physician communication such as:

Communication in Medical Care: Interaction Between Primary Care Physicians and Patients (Cambridge University Press, 2006)

Online Patient-Physician Communication: Benchmarking Physician Adoption (Adobe Acrobat Printable, 2006)

The Silent World of Doctor and Patient (The Johns Hopkins University Press, 2002)

Making the Patient Your Partner: Communication Skills for Doctors and Other Caregivers (Auburn House Paperback, 1997)

Communicating with Today's Patient: Essentials to Save Time, Decrease Risk and Increase Patient Compliance (Jossey-Bass, 2000)

Patient Education: A Practical Approach (McGraw-Hill/Appleton-Lang, 1996)

When and How to Get A Second Opinion

The Challenge

You may have tremendous faith in your physician, but you may also want to back up your physician's opinion with a second opinion. This is especially true if you have a serious condition that might require extensive, and expensive, diagnostics and surgery. Under these circumstances, you need to consider receiving a second opinion from another qualified physician that will either agree with the initial diagnosis and recommendation or lead you to consider alternatives. You would probably never get your car repaired or do expensive home improvements without receiving several opinions and bids, and this same care should be applied to your medical condition. Unfortunately, many people are used to doing what their physician is telling them without taking the necessary step of receiving a second opinion. A responsible physician will encourage you to get this second opinion, and may even be able to guide you to another physician qualified to assess your condition. The challenge is to recognize when a second opinion is needed, find a physician you can rely on to provide the second opinion and then using both opinions to form your own decisions regarding your condition. Getting a second opinion should be considered at almost all times, and, if properly used, can help you immensely in receiving the best treatment for you.

The Facts

The American Medical Association acknowledges it can be time consuming and expensive to get a second opinion and there are several factors to consider before going for a second medical opinion. They stress that having a minor condition may not be a good time for a second opinion, but list some times when a second opinion becomes necessary.

- Your physician recommends a second opinion. If your physician believes your condition is outside his or her area of expertise, he or she will probably refer you to a second opinion.
- Your physician recommends elective surgery. If the surgery is not an emergency, a second opinion may be required by your health insurance plan. You might

also want to learn if there are treatment options other than surgery that would produce acceptable to you.

- Your physician has not reached a diagnosis or the diagnosis is not clear. If your physician is having difficulty diagnosing your condition and you are not seeing any improvement after repeated visits to your physician, you might want to consider a second opinion.
- You have a very rare or very serious medical condition. Before undergoing treatment for such a condition, you may want to visit a specialist in the field to verify the diagnosis.
- You are told by your physician that nothing more can be done to help you.
- Your physician restricts the types of treatment you could receive.
- You have a feeling there is something wrong with the diagnosis or suggested treatment for your condition.

Getting a second opinion may be even more important when dealing with children's medical conditions, or pediatric conditions, since often children cannot always adequately explain their symptoms and are usually are not qualified to seek their own second opinion. Be aware that you will increase any possible discomfort or fear by seeking a second opinion for your child, but, if you carefully explain why you believe a second opinion is necessary and what it can show for the child's condition, you should have a better chance of getting your child a second opinion with a minimum of discomfort.

Just as there is for an initial physician visit, there are specific questions you should always ask when you are seeking a second opinion.

- Is there any chance the medical condition could have a different diagnosis?
- What alternative forms of treatment are available?
- What would happen to you if you do not have the treatment initially prescribed?
- What are the risks and potential side effects of the treatment?
- How will the treatment plan affect your health or overall quality of life?
- How long will the recovery period be from the treatment?
- If the second opinion differs from the initial one, why is that?

The Solutions

Before you seek a second opinion, make sure this will be paid for by your medical insurance, if you have any. Your insurance carrier or group may have very specific requirements on when and how to seek a second opinion. Some of these may involve having the physician who made the initial diagnosis and recommendation for treatment formally acknowledge the potential need for a second opinion. At the very least, you should determine if the physician you wish to consult for a second opinion is covered by your insurance plan, especially if the insurance is a PPO with a required list of physicians.

Whether you ask your physician for a referral for a second opinion or pursue a second opinion on your own, you should inform your first physician of your decision and who you plan on visiting. When you do so, you can ask about the procedures involved in having your medical records, including the results of any tests which have been performed, forwarded to the second physician.

Do not hesitate to inform your initial physician of your decision to have a second opinion and do not worry about insulting your physician with this decision. Your physician should not believe this decision by you means you do not trust him or her, and understand in some cases a second opinion is required. Do not be swayed if your physician disagrees with your decision to get a second opinion. This is not a decision that is up to him or her. You always have the option to get a second opinion by keeping your own health goals in mind and doing what needs to be done to make you feel comfortable about your medical care.

Once you have made the decision to seek a second opinion, you must go through the effort to do this in a responsible and productive way. Not taking the proper path in seeking a second opinion will only result in wasting your time and money. Here are some ways the American Heart Association recommends you seek a second opinion:

- Get a referral from your first physician for a second opinion.
- Talk to your friends or relatives about who has treated them for a similar condition and what their experience was.
- Acquire a list of approved physicians from your medical insurance company or your employer's health plan administrator.
- Contact your local medical society either by phone or by looking up their specific Website.
- Refer to the American Medical Directory, Directory of American Specialists or other medical professional directories. These materials should be available from your local library.

It is never too late to get a second opinion. Even if you have begun receiving treatment recommended from the initial physician, you can still get a second opinion to make sure you are receiving the proper treatment. In most cases, it is better to get a second opinion soon after the initial diagnosis is made, but this not a hard and fast rule. The only exception to this is if you have already had surgery.

If you are having difficulty in acquiring your records of your tests and diagnosis from the initial physician, or if the physician you are consulting for a second opinion wants to conduct further tests, you may need to go through the effort and expense of having additional diagnostic procedures. Again, you should check with your medical insurance to find out what additional tests will be paid for. In many cases, the best way to make sure your second physician receives your current records is to obtain a copy of them and hand-deliver them to the second physician consultation when you arrive for your first appointment.

Just as you would for an important visit to your initial physician, you should bring somebody along with you when you receive a second opinion. You may be in a mental state where you are not hearing the important information properly and a fresh set of ears may note things you might miss. Also, take notes of what is discussed during a second opinion consultation.

The Resources

Visit the following Websites for more information on getting a medical second opinion:

Medem, *www,medem.com*

About Pediatrics, *www.about.com*

American Heart Association, *www.heart.org*

Swedish Covenant Hospital, *www.swedish.org*

Web MD, *www.webmd.com*

Cancer Guide, *www.cancerguide.org*

Centers for Medicare/Medicaid, *www.cms.hhs.gov*

Several books can be very helpful in learning about getting a medical second opinion such as:

Second Opinions: Eight Clinical Medical Dramas (Penguin, 2001)

Second Opinion: Your Medical Alternatives (Linden Press, 1981)

AIDS: A Second Opinion (Seven Stories Press, 2001)

American Medical Association Complete Guide to Your Children's Health (Random House, 1998)

The Secrets of Medical Decision Making: How to Avoid Becoming a Victim of the Health Care Machine (Loving Healing Press, 2005)

American Medical Association Guide to Talking to Your Doctor (Wiley, 2001)

Section Two:

Therapy and Drug Treatments

10

Advances in Treating Cancer

The Challenge

Cancer, after heart disease, is the biggest killer disease throughout the world. Cancer is non-discriminatory and can attack people of all races and ethnic groups with equally lethal consequences. It can affect children, adults and seniors with the same speed. There are very few organs or body systems that are immune from cancers. People justifiably greet the news they have cancer with a mixture of fear and apprehension. But, over the last few decades, and continuing today, they can also face the illness with much hope. Physicians have become increasingly sophisticated in identifying cancers. New methods of treatment and surgery have helped make many cancers very curable and keep them from recurring. The process of healing may not be always pleasant, but the results are very encouraging in the continuing fight against this deadly illness. The challenge for the patient is to identify what could be warning signs of different types of cancer, get a diagnosis as soon as possible and find a regimen of treatment that can either cure the disease or put it into a stage of remission when it will present the least amount of concern or further treatment for the patient over the long haul. With the proper knowledge and appropriate choices, fighting cancer becomes a battle that can be won and the future points to even more advances.

The Facts

There are several warning signs that indicate the possibility of having a cancer, but the only way to determine cancerous tissues is by visiting your primary care physician and indicating your concerns over a medical condition. You should be even more aware of the possibility of developing cancer if you have a family history of the disease. Depending on the findings of a physical examination and initial tests by a primary care physician, you may be referred to a cancer specialist known as an oncologist. Often an oncologist is associated with a special clinic or hospital facility. The oncologist will conduct further tests and then determine a method of treatment that will meet the needs of your condition with the aim of eliminating the cancerous tissues and keeping them from spreading to other organs.

While researchers can point to certain environmental factors or lifestyle choices that may promote the development of cancer, the truth is no one really understands what causes cancer and why it affects some people but not others. One of the more promising methods in determining whether you may be at risk to develop cancer is to test your DNA for certain genetic indicators for the possibility you could be at risk. This does not mean you have the disease, only that you may have an increased likelihood to develop the condition and should pay extra attention to potential physical symptoms. The findings may also spur you to visit your physician more often for physicals or to check out areas of concern. The reliability of DNA testing for the possibility of cancer has been found to be very high and should not be taken lightly.

One of the difficulties in dealing with cancer is that, unlike other bacterial or even viral diseases, the cancer does not simply infect other cells. Rather the cancer cells take over the cells and order them to not only become cancerous but to spread the disease. Researchers are still not clear on how this process occurs, but it makes the disease especially difficult to understand and to treat. It also means there is a far greater likelihood that the disease can recur even after treatments or surgery have seemed to initially eliminate it. Unfortunately, once you have had cancer, you may get it again, but you can still have the same options in successfully dealing with it.

The Solutions

It is always a good idea to report any suspected disease conditions to your primary care physician for evaluation as soon as possible, but it is even more important with cancer. You have probably heard this many times, but the sooner you discover the presence of a cancerous condition, the better the chance you can isolate the condition and successfully treat it. Any suspicion that you may have cancer must be investigated immediately.

Cancer carries with it a heavy psychological burden that may not be equaled by any other condition. Cancer patients know that just because they have initially beat the condition, that it may not recur or have spread unknown to other parts of the body. This feeling of always being in danger from a medical condition can have far-reaching effects on a patient's quality of life and may lead to an unnecessary curtailment of certain activities because of the fear of the cancer recurring. This is unique from most medical conditions that can be treated and considered cured for good. For example, once you have an appendix removed, it is not going to grow back or present any other problems. The same cannot be said for cancer.

Physicians and therapists have long understood the psychological aspects of dealing with the disease and have created many support mechanisms to help patients understand what has happened to them, what to expect and how to deal with life post-cancer. These materials are disseminated online, made available in literature in the physician's office or through professional journals. Another excellent way to help cancer patients cope with the aftermath of cancer is to participate in group support sessions of fellow cancer survivors. Led by a professional therapist, in some cases also a cancer survivor, these group sessions allow post-cancer patients to express their fears, knowledge and concern and receive valuable practical information and emotional support to help deal with life without cancer. Some groups are of a general nature regarding cancer, others may be specific to cancer suffered by larger groups, such as breast cancer, colon cancer, prostate cancer and skin cancer. They are usually made available or offered through the oncology clinic for cancer patients.

There are many methods of dealing with cancers, with more options becoming available on a yearly basis. The idea is to provide effective treatment in the least uncomfortable method possible. They are usually designed to build on each other, with the oncologist starting with the least intrusive method and moving on to other stronger methods that may eventually mean surgery. The most common methods currently available for treating cancer are:

- Biologic therapy works by helping the immune system to function better by using naturally occurring substances to fight the cancer.
- Bone marrow transplants uses donated marrow from compatible sources, often a close family member and may include peripheral blood stem cell and cord blood transplants.
- Chemotherapy uses strong dosages of drugs to fight the cancerous cells and kill them, and carries significant side effects such as nausea, weakness and hair loss during the treatment.
- Complementary and alternative methods, sometimes called holistic medicine, seeks non drug and surgery methods to fight cancer.
- Radiation therapy uses powerful directed x-rays or radioactive pellets in the body to attack the cancerous area as accurately as possible. Like chemotherapy, radiation therapy can also cause some debilitating side effects.
- Gene therapy is cutting edge therapy that is designed to boost the immune system and improve the body's natural ability to fight cancer.
- Hormone therapy is similar to chemotherapy in using natural or synthetic hormones to shrink cancerous tumors.
- Photodynamic therapy, PDT, is a novel approach to fighting cancer by exposing a photosensitive drug to specific wavelengths of light to kill the cancer cells.
- Proton therapy is a form of radiation therapy that is showing great promise.
- Surgery is the ultimate cancer treatment that physically removes the cancerous and surrounding tissues when possible.
- Targeted therapies uses drugs to target specific pathways in the growth and development of cancerous tumors.
- Vaccine therapies is one of the most complex topics in modern cancer therapy and is a rapidly changing and evolving method of treatment.
- Biofusion therapy uses fused cells to kill cancers, stimulate immune responses or repair damaged tissues. It is still undergoing development by health facilities such as the Mayo Clinic.

The Resources

Visit the following Websites for more information on advances in cancer treatments:

Oncolink, *www.oncolink.com*

Senior Journal, *www.seniorjournal.com*

Mayo Clinic, *www.mayoclinic.org*

Country Doctor, *www.countrydoctor.co.uk*

National Cancer Institute, *www,cancer.gov*

American Cancer Society, *www.cancer.org*

Live Science, *www.livescience.com*

Several books can be very helpful in learning about advances in cancer treatments such as:

The Cancer Treatment Revolution: How Smart Drugs and Other New Therapies are Renewing Our Hope and Changing the Face of Medicine (Wiley, 2007)

Your Breast Cancer Treatment Handbook: Your Guide to Understanding the Disease (Unknown, 2004)

After Cancer Treatment: Heal Faster, Better, Stronger (Johns Hopkins University Press, 2006)

Outsmart Your Cancer: Alternative Non-Toxic Treatments that Work (Thoughtworks Publishing, 2004)

Understanding Cancer: A Patient's Guide to Diagnosis, Prognosis and Treatment (Johns Hopkins University Press, 1998)

Cancer—Step Outside the Box (Infinity 510 Squared Partners, 2006)

11

New Methods of
Treating Breast Cancer

The Challenge

Breast cancer is one of the most treatable forms of cancer with one of the highest rates of recovery if the disease is detected early. The emphasis on treating breast cancer over the last 20 years has been using regular physician visits, self-examinations and periodic mammograms to detect the condition. Also, it is now far less likely that a physician or oncologist, a cancer specialist, will use radical surgery to remove a breast and surrounding tissue rather than simply removing a malignant lump without further surgery. Lately there have been even more advances in the detection and treatment of breast cancers that make controlling the disease easier and far less uncomfortable for the patient. The challenge is to be aware of what these advances are, finding physicians who are prepared to explore these advances and having a realistic view of what these alternatives can provide.

The Facts

Some forms of cancer may be traced to lifestyle factors such as diet, smoking or excessive consumption of alcohol. Breast cancer does not usually show a cause and effect based on lifestyle or environmental factors. In many cases, the likelihood of breast cancer increases with a family history of breast cancer. Also, breast cancer can affect younger patients as well as older women.

One of the newer developments in the detection and classification of breast cancer is called TNM staging. This staging takes into account the size of the tumor, how the lymph glands or nodes are affected and whether the tumor has spread anywhere else. Determining the stage helps the breast cancer specialist to decide the best treatment for you. Physicians will also treat breast cancer depending on its grade. The TNM system for staging is used throughout the world. The name comes because the procedure separately but simultaneously assessing the size of the tumor (T), the nodes (N) and the metastases (M). This system is considered more accurate than the previously used number staging for breast cancer.

Often women will avoid breast examinations because they fear the results will mean radical surgery that will remove a breast and, possibly, the surrounding tissues. This is strongly tied into the issues of self-image and sexuality and how these will be affected by having a breast removed. Physicians are more and more dealing with the emotional impact of breast surgery and explanation of alternatives to encourage women to undergo early detection.

Besides the staging of your cancer, the outlook for treatment of breast cancer will also depend on the grade of the cancer. This is determined by examining the cancerous cells from a breast tumor under a microscope. The more normal the cells look, the lower the grade. Breast cancer has three grades: grade one is low grade, grade two is intermediate grade and grade three is high grade. High grade cancers may be faster growing and more likely to spread.

Beyond staging and grading there are other factors your physician or oncologist will consider when deciding on a method of treatment. These include whether you have gone through menopause, type of cancer you have, various tests on your cancer cells and your overall general health. The tests determine whether your cancer cells have hormone receptors such as estrogen and progesterone receptors. Many breast cancers are stimulated to grow by these female sex hormones. The results of these tests may determine whether you are likely to respond to hormone therapy.

Another test for breast cancer is called Her2. This test will help determine if your cancer will respond to the relatively new treatment of biological therapy known as trastuzumab or Herceptin. Your breast cancer will respond to Herceptin if you test strong positive for the protein of Her2.

The Solutions

Like most forms of cancer, the first step in effective treatment is to detect the illness as soon as possible. Women are encouraged to do regular self-examinations, with methods described by the American Cancer Society at *www.cancer.org*. Women, especially those with higher genetic risk factors should make yearly visits to their Primary Care Physicians for an examination that includes evaluating any possible lumps in the breast. Finally, women have a mammogram at least once every two years. This procedure is mildly uncomfortable and uses a diagnostic machine to compress the breast and examine the interior structure for any signs of potential lumps. Older women and those with higher risk factors may want to receive a mammogram on a yearly basis.

Under the TNM staging system a number is attached to the T rating from one to three indicating the size of the tumor. The one to three number system is also used to describe to what extent the cancer has impacted the surrounding lymph nodes. Finally the M rating is either zero for no sign of cancer spread to M1 where the cancer has spread to another part of the body not including the breast and lymph nodes under the arm. Under this system a tumor, for example, might be described as T2 N0 and M0 indicating a single tumor two to five centimeters across, no evidence of spread to any lymph nodes and no evidence of spread beyond the breast.

Determining breast cancer stages and grades predict survival rates from the cancer and what type of treatment may be needed. Early breast cancers less than two centimeters across with no cancer and low or intermediate grade will indicate a woman who might have at least an 85 percent chance of living ten years or more after diagnosis.

Choosing treatment for breast cancer where clinical trials are taking place means you will tend to do better. These cancer clinics usually have the best concentration of expertise. You may be able to take part in free trials of experimental treatment procedures that could be very successful. Physicians for a clinical trial procedure will probably monitor your condition more closely. Good attitudes are vital in treating cancer and you may have more confidence receiving treatment at a special facility, aiding in the healing process.

Depending on the nature, staging and grading of your breast cancer, there are several forms of treatment that are most commonly practiced and constantly being refined:

- Surgery either removing a lump or the entire breast;
- radiotherapy using concentrations of X-rays to kill the cancerous cells;
- hormone therapy using replacement female hormones to shrink tumors;
- chemotherapy using a mixture of toxic chemicals to destroy cancer cells and
- experimental biological treatments such as Herceptin.

Your physician may use one of these methods or a combination of several to treat your breast cancer depending on the cancer.

If you have no treatment choice for your cancer except to have a mastectomy you may choose to undergo breast reconstruction surgery afterwards. This surgery will help reshape the breast rather than rely on more clumsy prosthetics.

Over the last decade there has been a growing movement to look for alternative cancer treatments that do not involve radiation, drugs or surgery. These are sometimes referred to as holistic treatments and may include meditation, acupuncture, relaxation techniques and herbal medicines including flaxseed and black cohosh. While there is no definitive clinical evidence that holistic treatments will effectively treat cancer, there is surely subjective evidence that these treatments can work.

You have new choices in different types of advanced, yet traditional treatments. Partial breast radiation following surgery is a welcome alternative to the usual six weeks of radiation treatment usually prescribed for post-operation. A donut mastectomy removes less tissue, as well as skin-sparing or nipple-sparing mastectomy. Finally, oncologists are experimenting with forms of chemotherapy that attack only the cancer area and do not have the same range of side effects to the entire body. Some oncologists are using neoadjuvant chemotherapy to treat the cancer prior to surgery rather than afterwards.

The Resources

Visit the following Websites for more information on advances in breast cancer treatment:

American Cancer Society, *www.cancer.org*

Seattle Cancer Care Alliance, *www.seattlecca.org*

Cancer Research UK, *www.cancerhelp.org.uk*

National Cancer Center, *www.cancer.gov*

Breast Cancer Center, *www.breastcancer.org*

National Breast Cancer Foundation, *www.nationalbreastcancer.org*

Several books can be very helpful in explaining new treatments for breast cancer such as:

Your Breast Cancer Treatment Handbook: Your Guide to Understanding the Disease, Treatments, Emotions and Recovery from Breast Cancer (Unknown, 2004)

Take Charge of Your Breast Cancer: A Guide to Getting the Best Possible Treatment (Owl Books, 2002)

New Choices: The Latest Options in Treating Breast Cancer (Dodd Mead, 1985)

The Breast Cancer Book: What You Need to Know to Make Informed Decisions (Yale University Press, 2005)

Breast Cancer Basics and Beyond: Treatments, Resources, Self-Help, Good News, Updates (Hunter House, 2005)

Coping with Breast Cancer: A Practical Guide to Understanding, Treating and Living with Breast Cancer (Avery, 1998)

12

New Methods of Treating Lung Cancer

The Challenge

Lung cancer used to be considered a death sentence. Anyone diagnosed with the disease had a limited number of treatment options beyond radical surgery that may or may not have solved the cancer problem. Lung cancer also was more likely to spread into surrounding tissues and lymph nodes. Now, however, lung cancer is being seen as more treatable with a higher rate of cure than before. Also, many environmental and lifestyle factors have been identified as being primary causes of lung cancer and can be successfully avoided, thus limiting the potential for acquiring lung cancer. Like other cancers, a key component in treating the disease is in identifying its presence as soon as possible. The challenge for anyone concerned about lung cancer is identifying risk factors in their lives, eliminating those factors, undergoing early detection techniques and finding methods of treatment that can address the disease with the least amount of invasiveness and discomfort.

The Facts

Unlike many forms of cancer, researchers have linked the development of lung cancer to various identifiable lifestyle elements and environmental factors.

- smoking tobacco products;
- the use of drugs that are smoked such as marijuana;
- high exposure to particulates such as coal dust and
- exposure to friable asbestos containing materials whose fibers can be inhaled and trapped in the lining of the lungs.

There is a staging for lung cancer that basically rates how far the disease has progressed and what impact it has had on surrounding tissues including lymph nodes. There are different staging systems for lung cancer. The most common staging system groups lung cancers into one of four groups, or stages one through four, depending on how far the cancer has progressed. Depending on whether the lung cancer is small cell or large cell, the staging rating can be different.

The type of treatment for lung cancer chosen by your oncologist will depend on several factors: the type of lung cancer you have, where the cancer is within the lung, your overall health, whether and how much the cancer has spread and the results of various blood tests.

Because new treatments for lung cancer are very specific, doctors are being careful to use them only on patients who are likely to respond to them. There has been just as much research in advance lung cancer diagnostics as there has been for treatment procedures. Much of this research has involved identifying biological signatures or biomarkers that help guide treatment options. One technique used for this is gene expression profiling using DNA analysis looking for specific genetic changes or mutations. Another test is used to measure the number of EGFR gene copies in a tumor sample. This is called fluorescence in situ hybridization (FISH) and patients with a higher gene copy number are called FISH-positive. FISH-positive patients may react better to EGFR inhibitor therapies.

The Solutions

You can take preventive actions to prevent the development of lung cancer.

- Stop smoking.
- Avoid dusty environments where particulates may be present in heavy concentrations or, if you have to work in these environments, make sure they are properly ventilated.
- If necessary wear proper respiratory protection when working in dusty environments or with asbestos containing materials. This respiratory protection should not simply be a dust mask. Many dust particles and fibers can penetrate these masks. Instead, use respirators with high efficiency particulate airway (HEPA) masks that offer better protection.

Understanding the staging for small cell lung cancer is relatively simple. These can be limited diseases and extensive disease. This use of only two stages for small cell lung cancer is because this type of cancer has been shown to spread faster. In fact, most physicians will assume small cell lung cancer has spread to some extent even if they cannot immediately see the evidence of the spreading. The two stages for small cell lung cancer are:

- Limited disease meaning the cancer can only be seen in one lung, in nearby lymph nodes or in fluid that surrounds the lung, called pleural effusion and
- extensive disease meaning the cancer has spread outside the lung to the chest or to other parts of the body.

Non-small cell cancer does not spread as quickly or extensively as small cell lung cancer and is divided into four stages:

- **Stage One means the cancer is localized with no cancer in any lymph nodes.** Stage One non-small cell cancer is further divided into 1A and 1B. Stage

1A means the tumor is small. Stage 1B means the tumor is larger than three centimeters across or is growing in the main bronchus, the main lung. Stage 1B includes cancers that have spread into the inner covering of the lung or are responsible for a partial collapse of the affected lung.

- **Stage Two is divided into Stage 2A and Stage 2B.** Stage 2A means the cancer is small but has spread to the lymph nodes closest to the affected lung. Stage 2B means the cancer in the lung is larger than three centimeters across and there is cancer in the lymph nodes nearest the affected lung, or the cancer is not in the lymph nodes but has spread into the chest wall, the outer covering of the lung, the muscle at the bottom of the chest cavity or the outer covering of the heart.
- **Stage Three is divided into Stage 3A and Stage 3B.** Stage 3A means there is cancer in the nodes further away from the affected lung or there is cancer only in nodes nearest to the affected lung but has also spread to the chest wall or the lung covering, pleura, or middle of the chest, mediastinum. Stage 3B means there is cancer in the nodes on the other side of the chest or above either collarbone, there is more than one tumor in the affected lobe of the lung, the tumor has grown into another major structure in the chest or there is a fluid collection around the lung that contains cancer cells, a malignant pleural effusion.

Small cell lung cancer is mostly treated with chemotherapy because it has likely already spread to other areas of the body and is non-operable. Non-small cell lung cancer can be treated individually or with a combination of surgery, chemotherapy or radiotherapy.

There have been several new developments in the treatment of lung cancer with more on the way depending on the results of clinical trials.

- Percutaneous radiofrequency ablation or RFA uses a needle through the skin and into the lung tumor. Then radio waves are passed through the needle and heat the cancer cells until they are killed.
- New combinations of chemotherapy are being developed that cause fewer and less debilitating side effects. Also researchers are looking for drugs that will work if a patient develops a resistance to the chemotherapy.
- Genes altered by the cancer can be corrected by newer forms of biological drugs.
- Drugs are being used that interrupt the angiogenesis of lung cancers, destroying their blood vessels vital for tumor growth.
- Photo dynamic therapy (PDT) uses light to treat cancer.
- Cryotherapy uses a freezing probe to kill cancer and free airway blockages caused by the cancer.
- Epidermal growth factor receptor (EGFR) inhibitors interrupt cancer's ability to divide and grow. Vascular endothelial growth factor (VEGF) inhibitors are used in a similar manner to interrupt tumor blood supply.

The Resources

Visit the following Websites for more information on advances in lung cancer treatment:

American Cancer Society, *www.cancer.org*

University of Maryland Medical Center, *www.umm.edu*

Cancer Research UK, *www.cancerhelp.org.uk*

Medical News, *www.medicalnewstoday.com*

Patient Health International, *www.patienthealthinternational.com*

American Lung Association, *www.lungusa.org*

Several books can be very helpful in explaining new treatments for lung cancer such as:

Lung Cancer: A Guide to Diagnosis and Treatment (Addicus Books, 2001)

Lung Cancer: Myths, Facts Choices—and Hope (W.W. Norton and Company, 2003)

Multimodality Treatment of Lung Cancer (Informa Healthcare, 2000)

Progress and Perspectives in the Treatment of Lung Cancer (Springer, Verlag, Telos, 1999)

Biology and Management of Lung Cancer (Springer, 1983)

Lung Cancer Advances in Research and Treatment (Churchill Livingstone, 1985)

13

New Methods of Treating Prostate Cancer

The Challenge

Prostate cancer is one of the most common forms of cancer for men to experience. It is cancer of small gland located in the groin area. The urinary and sexual functions of a man can be severely affected by a cancerous prostate. A prostate examination involving physical manipulation of the gland is usually the first step in determining the possible presence of prostate cancer. Depending on the results of this examination, a physician may want to use imaging and blood tests to confirm that the prostate gland is cancerous. Often times, an enlarged prostate, which is not cancerous can be mistaken for a cancerous prostate since the symptoms are largely the same. This is one reason why a physical examination is recommended for any man who believes he is experiencing prostate problems. Another fallacy is that prostate cancer only affects older men. Younger men may be less likely to develop prostate cancer, but that is not impossible, so men of any age experiencing pain or difficulty urinating should see their physicians as soon as possible. The challenge is when to recognize common symptoms of prostate problems, knowing what to ask a physician regarding the condition and taking the proper actions in confirming the condition and treating it. With the proper knowledge, a man can effectively deal with prostate cancer and avoid lasting physical harm or early death.

The Facts

Staging measurement determines the location of the cancer. Staging is rated from T1 to T4. Staging is often considered the least accurate measure of the extent of the cancer, with the biggest area of inaccuracy being for the T1 or T2 of the cancer.

One should expect that various specialists are going to recommend various types of treatment for prostate cancer depending on their areas of specialization. In a sense, this is like shopping for a car where each salesperson is promoting their brand of cars as the right way to go. A urologist may push a surgical solution, an oncologist may recommend using high-grade and targeted radiation. The best way to make a decision regarding possible prostate treatment is to be as informed as possible on the condition and what may be best for you.

A normal-sized prostate is about the size of a walnut and is surrounded by a capsule similar to a shell around an egg. The urethra, a tube, runs through the middle of the prostate and drains urine from the bladder out of the penis. About two thirds of the prostate gland is made up of normal cells and the remaining third is made up of the urethra.

Although it seems illogical, prostate cancer tends to spread to the bones rather than any other organs. In prostate cancer, it is occasionally possible for cancer spread, metastases, to be present even when the prostate tumor is relatively small. If the tumor appears to be very small, but a bone scan reveals there is cancer n the bones, he prostate cancer is at the higher level of Stage 4.

The Solutions

It is certainly tempting to concentrate immediately on starting some type of treatment as soon as you determine you have prostate cancer, but this is a mistake. Instead, you should be taking the time to become as familiar as possible with the nature of the disease, how it has been diagnosed and what the extent of the disease is in your body. This knowledge will help you determine your treatment and what type of physician can provide it.

One of the primary methods in determining possible prostate cancer is to measure PSA, an enzyme that is produced by either normal or cancerous prostate cells and secreted into the seminal fluid. Measuring PSA in a simple blood test, can help identify a prostate gland as possibly cancerous. The normal level of PSA for men aged 60 or less is 2.5 ng/ml. For older men the range is higher, 4.0 ng/ml. This is because the prostate enlarges and generates more PSA in older men. Men with cancerous prostate will often, but not always, have PSA levels that are elevated above the normal levels of 2.5 ng/ml or 4.0 ng/ml. The average level of PSA for men with cancerous prostates is 7.0 ng/ml.

Another score in determining the nature of a prostate cancer is the Gleason score. This score indicates how fast the cancer is growing. The Gleason score ranges from two to 10. The Gleason score is determined by doing a biopsy of the effected tissue and examining that tissue under a microscope.

To be truly considered cured of prostate cancer you must have absolutely no cancerous cells left in that area. This is usually achieved through major surgery called a radical prostatectomy. If the PSA is still more than 0.2 ng/ml following surgery, you are not fully cured. Approximately 15 percent of men will not be cured of prostate cancer after surgery. Cancer cell leakage can be missed or spread through lymph channels or tiny blood vessels not detectable with a microscope.

A radical prostatectomy means the removal of the prostate gland and must be done as major surgery under general anesthetic. It can have significant side effects in sexual activity and urination. Other options for treatment of prostate cancer are through various types of radiotherapy that use radiation to kill the cancerous cells in the prostate.

- A radioactive iodine prostate seed implant with an ultrasound machine;
- linear accelerator irradiation using either conformal beams or intensity modulated radiotherapy, IMRT, techniques and
- daily accelerator irradiation.

Knowing cure rates for prostate cancer is vital in deciding on a treatment. You do not want to be just treated for prostate cancer, you want to be cured of it by establishing a PSA level at or below 0.2 ng/ml. A good way to determine cure rates is to ask your physician about all the men he or she has treated ten years ago and how many of these have PSA 0.23 ng/ml today. There is no best way to cure cancer between a radical prostactemy, where the prostate is removed and radiation therapies. The treatment is an informed guess based on prior experience and test results. This means you must find a physician to treat your prostate condition who has had extensive experience in prostate cancer detection and treatment. You can determine this experience by asking hard questions of the physician and demanding detailed answers.

If you have low grade prostate cancer , your physician may recommend a watch and wait approach and see if any other symptoms develop. This is especially true with older patients who may live only to the point where the cancer begins exhibiting debilitating symptoms. The watch and wait eliminates enduring treatments that may cause side effects worse than symptoms from the cancer. If you have high-grade prostate cancer, it will almost certainly be recommended you have some type of treatment.

Besides the accepted treatments of radical prostatectomy and radiation, your physician may recommend you explore other treatment possibilities that are only now being pioneered. These include hormone therapy, brachytherapy that uses the implantation of radioactive seeds, chemotherapy for prostate cancer that has spread and cryotherapy that freezes the cancer tissue and kills it, high-frequency ultrasound that heats the affected area, photodynamic therapy that uses light to kill cancers, vaccine therapy and gene therapy using stem cells,

The Resources

Visit the following Websites for more information about treating prostate cancer:

American Cancer Society, *www.cancer.org*

National Prostate Cancer Coalition, *www.fightcancer.org*

American Urological Association, *www.auanet.org*

Prostate Cancer Foundation, *www.prostatecancerfoundation.org*

Cancer Guide: Prostate Cancer, *www.cancerguide.org/prostate*

Cancer Research, *www.cancerresearch.org*

Radiation Clinics of Georgia, *www.rcog.com*

Several books can be very helpful in learning about treatment for prostate cancer such as:

Prostate Cancer for Dummies (For Dummies, 2003)

Surviving Prostate Cancer Without Surgery (Roseville Books, 2005)

Prostate and Cancer: A Family Guide to Diagnosis, Treatment and Survival (Perseus Books Groups, 2003)

How I Survived Prostate Cancer, and So Can You: A Guide for Diagnosing and Treating Prostate Cancer (Health Education Literary Publisher, 1994)

The Prostate: A Guide for Men and the Women Who Love Them (Warner Books, 1997)

The First Year Prostate Cancer: An Essential Guide for the Newly Diagnosed (Marlowe & Company, 2005)

14

New Methods of Treating Colon Cancer

The Challenge

Colon cancer can cover a variety of conditions and be present in varying stages of development. Colon cancer is equally likely to strike women or men, and, while it usually is present at or beyond a certain age, it can strike anytime. Its presence can be indicated with some obvious physical symptoms and then confirmed through a colon examination and blood tests. It is easily detected and can be treated effectively. However, like many forms of cancer, this type of cancer can spread to surrounding tissues and lymph nodes causing problems that are potentially more severe of possibly life threatening than the original cancer. The challenge is to maintain awareness of what symptoms might indicate possible colon cancer, properly placing these conditions within the historical context of your overall health, clearly expressing your concerns to your physician, going through the discomfort of examination for colon cancer, following up to determine if the disease has spread and then deciding on an effective form of treatment. This type of cancer is very treatable, but must be caught and recognized early. Once you do so, you have a very good chance of detecting and curing the disease.

The Facts

One of the most common symptoms indicating you are suffering colon cancer is difficulty in having regular bowel movements and detecting some blood in the stool. These symptoms may be attributable to other factors, for example blood in the stool may be caused by bleeding hemorrhoids, but the only way to detect definitively if you are suffering from colon cancer you should receive a comprehensive physical examination.

Unlike with prostate cancer, women are just as likely to develop colon cancer as men and should be examined for the disease, especially if they believe they may be suffering from obvious symptoms that indicate the presence of colon cancer.

Most insurance plans will pay a large portion of the costs for testing for colon cancer, especially when the testing is ordered through a specialist after the recommendation of a primary care physician. This recommendation may be based on a specific condition noted by the patient or because of the age and risk factors for the patient. However, coverage for testing or screening for colon cancer is only reimbursed by Medicare at a fraction of what the procedure would cost. This is especially a problem because those who are most likely to develop colon cancer are older patients who are covered by Medicare benefits. Under new proposed legislation on a federal level, colorectal screening procedures would be exempt from the customary Medicare deductible requirement regardless of the outcome of the screening. The legislation also calls for Medicare to cover a preoperative visit or consultation before the screening or colonoscopy.

If colon cancer is detected early enough, it is highly curable. In fact, it is one of the most curable forms of cancer. Based on numbers from *www.cancer.org* and using standard staging ratings for the severity of the cancer the cure rates can be measured. In this system, Stage I means the cancer has spread beyond the innermost lining of the colon or rectum; Stage II means the cancer has spread outside the colon or rectum to nearby tissue; Stage III means the cancer has spread to nearby lymph nodes; Stage IV means the cancer has spread to other areas of the body and Recurrent Cancer means the cancer has come back after treatment. The survival rates are:

Colon Cancer Survival Rates

Stage	Survival Rates
I	93 percent
IIA	85 percent
IIB	72 percent
IIIA	83 percent
IIIB	64 percent
IIIC	44 percent
IV	8 percent

The Solutions

Although anybody of any age has the potential to develop colon cancer, the chances of you developing the disease increases if there is a history of colon cancer in your family. If so, your physician may be especially diligent about asking about any symptoms that might indicate the presence of colon cancer but also use a colonoscopy to look for any signs of cancer. Colonoscopies are usually recommended as part of a regular physical examination after a patient is 50 years old and then done periodically.

A colonoscopy is a relatively comfortable diagnostic procedure. It uses a sedative to gray out the patient, where the patient is not completely asleep but is drugged to the point where the procedure will not give undue discomfort and the patient will remain still during the procedure. The colonoscopy uses a thin tube inserted into the colon.

There is a camera at the end of the colonoscope to look for possible cancerous tissue. If any possible cancerous tissue is visually detected, the colonoscope can snip off a small portion of the tissue, retrieve it from the colon and allow it to examined in a laboratory for the presence of cancer cells. Alternatives to colonoscopy include blood sampling and testing and the testing of stool samples brought to the physician by the patient. The standard test, though, for colon cancer is the colonoscopy and is much more definitive than other methods.

Treatment for colon cancer involves three main types of procedures. Depending on the nature of the disease, two or more treatments may be recommended for a patient with colorectal cancers. Like other medical procedures, you should plan on getting two sets of opinions as to whether treatment is needed and what type of treatment you should consider. Be sure to take a careful look at the background and experience of the medical team treating your cancer. Here are the main types of treatment you can consider:

- Surgery is the main treatment for colon cancer. The surgery usually involves removal of the cancer and length of normal colon on either side of the cancer. The two ends of the colon are then sewn back together. Sometimes surgery for early-stage colon cancer can be done with minimally invasive procedures such as using a colonoscope or other instruments inserted into the colon via the anus. Specially trained nurses can help you manage your recovery from a colostomy or urostomy. Possible side effects of surgery include bleeding from the surgery, blood clots in the legs and damage to nearby organs during the surgery. If the colorectal cancer has spread to areas in the lungs, liver, ovaries or elsewhere in the abdomen, surgery might be needed to remove the cancers from these areas.
- Radiation therapy uses high-energy rays, such as x-rays, to kill or shrink cancer cells. The radiation may be administered from outside the body or from radioactive materials placed directly in the region of the tumor. Radiation may be used after surgery to kill residual cancer cells. Sometimes radiation is used for areas that are large or hard to get to by being used prior to the surgery to shrink the tumors. Radiation is especially recommended for patients who have had colorectal cancer that has attached to nearby organs or the lining of the abdomen. Side effects of radiation therapy include mild skin irritation, nausea, diarrhea, rectal or bladder irritation or fatigue. Sexual problems can also occur. The side effects usually go away after the radiation is received.
- Chemotherapy uses cancer-fighting drugs injected into a vein or given orally. The drugs enter the body mainstream and treat organs at some distance from the colon. Chemotherapy is often used after surgery to eliminate cancers that remain or have spread to the other organs such as the lymph nodes. Side effects from chemotherapy can be severe and include diarrhea, nausea and vomiting, loss of appetite, loss of hair, hand or foot rashes and swelling, mouth sores, increased infections, increased bleeding or bruising after minor injuries and severe fatigue. Most side effects will go away after treatment.

The Resources

Visit the following Websites for more information about treating colon cancer:

Kaiser Network, *www.kaisernetwork.org*

Healthlink, *www.healthlink.mcw.edu*

Cancer.org, *www.cancer.org*

Web MD, *www.webmd.com*

Hershey Medical Center, *www.hmc.psu.edu*

About Colon Cancer, *www.coloncancer.about.com*

Medicine Net, *www.medicinenet.com*

Several books can be very helpful in learning about treatment for colon cancer such as:

Everyone's Guide to Cancer Therapy 4th Edition (Andrews McMeel Publishing, 2002)

Colon Cancer & the Polyps Connection (De Capo, 2001)

Preventing and Treating Colon Cancer (Harvard Health Publications, 2001)

What to Do If You Get Colon Cancer: A Specialist Helps You Take Charge and Make Informed Choices (Wiley, 1997)

Understanding Colon Cancer (University Press of Mississippi, 2002)

Cancer Doesn't Have to Hurt: How to Conquer the Pain Caused by Cancer and Cancer Treatment (Hunter House, 1997)

15

New Methods of
Treating Skin Cancer

The Challenge

Skin cancer can often be ignored as simply a blemish or mole. In can be caused by heredity or exposure to environmental elements, such as excessive exposure to the sun. Whatever its cause, skin cancer can strike anybody of any age and is frequently a surprise condition that is found only during a thorough physical examination. Skin cancer may seem minor compared to other types of cancer such as lung cancer or breast cancer, but skin cancer can quickly turn into a very dangerous condition that can cause severe physical problems in a short amount of time. The challenge is to know what to look for that may constitute some form of skin cancer, how soon to visit your doctor and communicate your concern, what methods of diagnosis will be used and, if you are diagnosed with skin cancer, what are the latest treatments to combat the disease. Knowledge and early follow-up are essential to identifying a number of physical conditions and skin cancer is one of the most obvious examples of these requirements.

The Facts

One of the most significant causes of skin cancer is severe exposure to the sun. This is by people who work in the sun without proper skin covering or those who have spent their lives as sun worshipers, spending a lot of time sunning themselves at the beach, at a park or in a tanning bed.

Not all skin cancers are created equally. There are three main types of skin cancer that have to be dealt with in their own ways. Basal cell carcinomas and squamous cell carcinomas are slow developing and relatively easy to treat by physicians. The dangerous form of the disease is malignant melanoma, a fast-growing type of skin cancer that can spread very quickly and be difficult to treat.

Skin cancer may be perceived as a minor condition compared to other types of cancers but malignant melanomas is one of the most dangerous forms of cancer. If diagnosed too late, treatment methods may not be enough to stop the cancer. Squamous cell carcinomas grow very slowly and are not seen as dangerous and basal cell carcinomas barely grow at all. Even in advanced cases of basal cell carcinomas, treatments are usually successful.

Skin cancers are some of the most common encountered by consumers and physicians. Figures in the United Kingdom list an average of 6,000 cases of melanoma diagnosed every year and 62,000 cases of lesser dangerous cancers reported every year. This figure of 62,000 may be misleading since the cancers are slow-growing and may remain undiagnosed for some time, especially among older patients who may see the condition as normal aging spots. Roughly 75 percent of non-melanoma skin cancers are basal cell carcinomas and the others are squamous cell carcinomas.

Skin cancers can run in families. Some rare, inherited skin diseases can make people more sensitive to sunlight and more likely to acquire skin cancer. People who inherit pale, freckly skin are typically more susceptible to skin cancers. If you have a close relative who suffered from skin cancer, you can have almost twice the normal risk of getting the same type of skin cancer.

Depending on the severity and cosmetic damage from surgery for skin cancer, you may be referred to a plastic surgeon after treatment from a dermatologist. The plastic surgeon can help use tissue grafts and other techniques to rebuild the areas on the body affected by the surgery. Going through this additional surgery will depend on how you feel about your body image and what can be seen.

The Solutions

You must understand that skin cancer is not caused by exposure to all aspects of sunlight. Ultra violet rays, also caused by tanning sun beds, is an element of sunlight that can damage the DNA in skin cells. This damage may make a cell cancerous. Ultra violet, UV light, is classified as A, B and C. UVC is filtered out by the atmosphere and does not reach the skin. The original cause of sunburn and skin cancer was thought to be caused by UVB rays, but now UVA is also known to cause sunburn and skin cancer. Modern sun beds produce less UVA and sun creams are more effective in blocking out UVA rays. People who wear a UVA blocking cream may spend more time in the sun, and increase their risk of developing skin cancers.

More and more physicians are urging people to avoid certain behaviors and take actions that may limit their exposure to the potentially cancer-causing effects of prolonged exposure to the ultra violet rays of the sun.

- Wearing an effective sun screen on any skin that will have prolonged exposure to the ultra violet rays of the sun;
- covering up exposed areas such as the arms and legs and wearing a hat or cap with a brim that will help shield the face and
- limiting the time you are exposed to the sun by adding planned time in the shade to any solar exposure.

Although anybody with suspected skin cancer should consult their physicians immediately for an evaluation, there are factors in appearance and spreading that may tell your primary care physician what type of cancer you have.

- Most melanomas, the most dangerous type of skin cancer, occur on the head, neck, arms and back. They are usually very dark or black but can sometimes be light brown or even speckled. The surface is rough and usually raised. In early stages, melanomas can look like moles, but with a ragged outline or differing shades of color. Sometimes they may be bleeding, oozing or crusting. The most important thing to evaluate is whether the suspected areas change shape or color as they grow.
- Basal cell carcinomas usually occur on the face and start as small, pink, pearly or waxy spots. As they grow, the form a raised, flat spot with a rolled edge and may develop a crust. The next step in growth may be to bleed from the center and develop ulcers, called rodent ulcers.
- Squamous cell carcinomas usually occur on the arms and legs, head or neck. They are pink and irregular in shape, often with a hard, scaly or horny surface, or sometimes they can ulcerate. The edges are sometimes raised and the spots can be tender to the touch.

Minor surgery to remove the cancerous non-melanoma spots and some of the surrounding tissue will usually be effective against carcinomas. Melanomas are much more difficult to treat, surgery does not adequately do the job. A patient may have to look at chemotherapy and radiotherapy to be used on secondary tumors. This type of treatment of melanomas will prolong life but cannot provide a cure for the cancer. A key to any type of surgery is removing surrounding tissue from the affected area.

The most effective way to deal with skin cancers of any types is to get early detection of the disease. This is especially important in the fast-moving type of melanoma. A physician can recognize potential skin cancer and sample the tissue to determine if it is cancerous. How early the disease is detected will affect how the disease is treated and how effective that treatment may be.

A new type of treatment for skin cancer is called photodynamic therapy, or PDT. It is not recommended for squamous cell skin cancers. PDT using a cream is available for treatment and is best used in cases that may require a large amount of surgery. PDT is not as effective against deeper skin cancers, because light cannot penetrate far enough into the skin to activate the treatment.

Retinoids, chemicals similar to Vitamin A can be taken in tablet form or applied to the affected area in a cream. Another experimental method of treating skin cancer is using Interferon, a type of immunotherapy. Interferon stimulates the body's immune system to find and fight cancer cells.

If you believe you have some type of skin cancer, there are specific questions you should ask your physician.

- What stage is my skin cancer?
- How will the stage affect my treatment?
- What treatment is recommended?
- What other treatment choices do I have?
- Do I need to be hospitalized or can I be treated as an outpatient?
- What are the treatment side effects?
- Will the cancer come back?
- What should I do to protect my skin in the future?

The Resources

Visit the following Websites for more information about skin cancer:

American Cancer Society, *www.cancer.org*

AICR United Kingdom, *www.aicr.org.uk*

Cancer Help, *www.cancerhelp.org.uk*

MKMG, *www.mkmg.com*

Mayo Clinic, *www.mayoclinic.org*

Plastic Surgery, *www.plasticsurgery.org*

Skin Cancer Foundation, *www.skincancer.org*

Several books can be very helpful in learning about skin cancer such as:

Only Skin Deep? An Essential Guide to Effective Skin Cancer Programs and Treatments (iUniverse Inc., 2007)

100 Questions and Answers about Melanoma and Other Skin Cancers (Jones and Bartlett Publishers, Inc., 2003)

The Skin Cancer Answer: the Natural Treatment for Basal and Squamous Cell Carcinomas (Avery, 1998)

Cancer of the Skin (W.B. Saunders, 1991)

Quickfacts on Skin Cancer (American Cancer Society, 2007)

Sun Protection for Life: Your Guide to A Lifetime of Healthy & Beautiful Skin (New Harbinger Publications, 2005)

16

Advances in Treating Heart Conditions

The Challenge

Heart conditions are the number one cause of pain, suffering, hospitalization, changes in lifestyle and death for Americans, followed closely by cancer. However, unlike cancer which cannot be easily predicted until the disease manifests itself, physicians can identify heart risk factors and the early onset of possible heart conditions. This early warning capability vastly increases the likelihood that heart conditions can be detected before they cause major health problems and successfully treated through medication, changes in lifestyle, and, when absolutely necessary, surgery. Although the nature of the heart disease may range from atrial fibrillation to heart failure to stroke, a person with heart problems does not have to wait for something catastrophic to happen before seeking treatment. The challenge is to recognize heart risk factors, visiting a physician early enough to detect any potential heart problems and following through on the latest advances in treating heart disease. These advances can save your life and, at the very least, spare you the suffering caused by common heart conditions.

The Facts

Improper diet and lack of exercise are two of the most important risk factors in heart. Anyone over the age of 55 should closely monitor their numbers, meaning primarily their cholesterol levels. These levels can indicate conditions that can bring on heart problems. HDL is considered good cholesterol and should be over 60. LDL is the bad cholesterol and should be below 100. Other numbers related to cholesterol that should be monitored include triglycerides and blood glucose levels. These numbers can also indicate possible diabetes.

Knowing your family history is vital in leading a physician to diagnose heart disease. Heart disease can be considered a family disease. If your immediate family, including your father, mother, grandparents and aunts and uncles, suffered from some type of heart condition, it is more likely you will incur these types of conditions in your own life. A family history of heart disease is not a guarantee you will suffer from heart disease, but it can be a red light for physicians to pay attention to your heart and use diagnostic techniques such as stress tests and angiograms to detect possible heart problems.

A catastrophic heart condition is heart failure where the heart muscle can no longer pump enough blood to the body. Patients suffering from heart failure are unable to carry on any type of daily activities, even simple walking around. This is a debilitating condition that will only get worse as time goes by.

The most common symptoms of heart disease are shortness of breath, shoulder pain that radiates all the way down to the fingertips, epigastric pain, a constant feeling of fatigue and loss of sleep at night. Physicians caution that not all potential symptoms indicate heart problems. For example, a patient who has suffered from periodic chest pain since childhood is probably not suffering from a heart condition. However, if symptoms occur shortly after any type of exertion, this is a more common indicator of potential heart disease.

Another common heart condition is a stroke, normally caused by a blood vessel blockage that prevents proper blood flow to the brain. This lack of blood may cause a patient to lose feeling or movement in one side of the body and can be a frightening experience.

Another common form of heart disease is atrial fibrillation (AFIB). AFIB is a severe interruption of the natural rhythm of the heartbeat resulting in a chaotic activity of the heart. Patients can feel their heart rates dropping then increasing rapidly. AFIB can cause heart attacks and result in extreme discomfort for the patient.

Chest pain experienced from normal exertion that can feel debilitating is called angina. Angina patients can be treated by medications that relax blood vessels and improve blood flow. Similar medications can be used to treat chronic high blood pressure or regulate and slow down the rate of the heart.

The Solutions

A growing diagnostic tool in detecting possible heart conditions is genetic testing. Genetic testing involves taking a blood sample and looking for genetic markers that indicate the possibility of some, but not all, types of potential heart disease. This genetic testing is usually justified if a patient has a family history of heart disease. Genetic testing has been successfully used for many years to indicate the possible development of cancer, and is just now being used for some types of heart disease.

The most common form of battling cholesterol problems that can cause heart disease is to change diet, increase exercise and use drugs to reduce LDL cholesterol. A new type of cholesterol treatment is starting to show promise. The treatment, called EXPLORER, which combines two common types of cholesterol treating drugs into one drug therapy. Preliminary studies indicate the EXPLORER treatment can reduce LDL cholesterol in high-risk patients by 70 percent.

Physicians do have some choices in treating heart failure. They can install pacemakers, or even more complicated ventricular assist devices (VADs) that stimulate the heart muscle and require the patient to carry a portable battery to power the device. The ultimate solution in treating heart failure is to do a heart transplant, which have become relatively common and reliable over the last 20 years.

Any patient who thinks he or she is having heart problems should visit their primary care physician (PCP) as soon as possible for a preliminary evaluation. The PCP, based on that evaluation, can recommend the patient undergo further testing or visit a cardiologist for a full evaluation. A patient experiencing immediate and debilitating pain or shortness of breath should visit an Emergency Room or call an ambulance as soon as possible.

Many hospitals have stroke teams in place to handle potential strokes. The initial care involves using drugs to eliminate the blockage. Newer, cutting edge techniques in treating strokes involve mechanical thrombolosyis and balloon angioplasty to dissolve and remove a blood clot. A fascinating new technology is using bat saliva to treat stroke patients. Bat saliva contains a naturally-occurring thrombolythic element which can dissolve blood clots.

AFIB, a common form of heart disease from irregular heart activity, can be treated in several ways. Physicians usually start with the least intrusive form of treatment and work their way up from there.

Medications;
1. atrial ablations which uses radio frequencies to cauterize the heart by heating up the heart to create a scar which can easy AFIB symptoms;
2. cryoablation is similar to atria ablation except it freezes the heart to minus 70 degrees centigrade to treat AFIB. Cryoablation will cause fewer side effects than normal atrial ablation and
3. Maze surgery that actually opens the chest in a procedure called a sternotomy. This allows surgeons to access the heart and use scarring to treat AFIB.

Modern treatment techniques for heart conditions are emphasizing using non-invasive or less invasive procedures as often as possible. Hospitalization for heart disease fell 11 percent from 2002 to 2005, according to researchers in Michigan. Instead of heart bypass surgeries, physicians are relying more on angioplasty and arterial stents. This results in patients spending less time in a hospital and using outpatient facilities. This availability helps heart patients get past their fear of having their chests opened and may prompt them to more quickly seek treatment.

A promising new treatment in heart disease is the use of cell therapy. Depending on future research, this cellular therapy may involve the use of human stem cells to regrow damaged heart tissue. Currently cells used in treating heart disease are acquired from autologous donors' (donors who are also the recipient of cell therapy) skeletal muscle. Stem cells from autologous peripheral blood and bone marrow can also be used.

Once a patient has undergone heart treatment and are sent home or are treated through lifestyle changes for heat conditions, they are instructed to follow basic guidelines.

- Use up at least as many calories as you take in. Monitor your normal calorie intake and plan activities or exercises. This means at least 30 minutes a day of moderate exertion. This can also help you lose weight.
- Eat a variety of nutritious foods and avoid the junk: eat vegetables and fruits, whole-grain foods and fish.
- Avoid fat by eating lean meat, consume less hydrogenated vegetable oils, salt, sugary foods and moderate alcohol intake.
- Stop smoking, and, when possible avoid second-hand smoke.

The Resources

Visit the following Websites for more information on advances in heart treatment:

American Heart Association, *www.americanheart.org*

Scripps News, *www.scippsnews.com*

John Muir Health, *www.johmuirhealth.com*

Federal Drug Administration, *www.fda.gov*

Ohio State University Medical Center, *www.osumc.edu*

University of Connecticut, *www.uconn.edu*

Several books can be very helpful in explaining new heart treatments such as:

Reversing Heart Disease: A Vital New Program to Help Prevent, Treat and Eliminate Cardiac Problems Without Surgery (Warner Books, 2002)

What to Eat if You Have Heart Disease: Nutritional Therapy for the Prevention and Treatment of Cardiovascular Disease (McGraw-Hill, 1998)

Coronary Hearth Disease: A Guide to Diagnosis and Treatment (Addicus Books, 2002)

The Expert Guide to Beating Heart Disease: What You Absolutely Must Know (Collins, 2005)

You Can Beat Heart Disease (Better Life Press, 2000)

Treatment of Heart Disease (Gower Medical Publishing, 1992)

17

Using Advanced Antibiotics

The Challenge

More and more we are hearing about infectious diseases that are becoming resistant to standard antibiotics. This resistance is prompting researchers and physicians to look at alternatives in advanced antibiotics. This means using methods of treating infections and infectious diseases that allow physicians to treat without overtreating and avoid using antibiotics that can build up their own resistance. The challenge is to identify what diseases can effectively be treated with these advanced antibiotics, what are the choices available, what are the clear benefits and what are the side effects to be concerned about. With proper knowledge and close consultation with your physician, you can play an active role in using antibiotic treatment and take full advantage of what are justly considered to be the wonder drugs of the last two centuries.

The Facts

Antibiotics were considered wonder drugs when they were developed in the early part of the 20th century. They were developed to treat certain diseases caused by bacteria. Antibiotics traditionally have little or no effect on diseases caused by a virus, such as influenza. The first major antibiotic developed was penicillin, which was discovered by accident by chemist Alexander Fleming. Early antibiotics were formed from living organisms. Later antibiotics were created chemically to treat bacterial diseases and infections. A pioneer in developing chemical-based antibiotics was Dr. Paul Ehrlich. Ehrlich originally developed his antibiotics to treat patients with syphilis, which up until then was virtually untreatable. Physicians prior to the development of antibiotics relied on what were called sulfa drugs. These drugs were only intermittently effective and often caused more problems than they solved.

Antibiotics showed their worth during World War II, saving the lives of thousands of wounded soldiers who had to undergo battlefield surgery. Prior to the use of antibiotics, such as penicillin, these soldiers would have died due to infections from their wounds and emergency surgery.

Many potentially dangerous infections can occur during a hospital stay. These include pneumonia and sepsis, complicated skin and skin structure infections. This serious infection has a mortality rate of around 40 percent and a death toll of about 1,400 hospital deaths. In fact, disabled actor Christopher Reeve died from complications due to skin infections caused by prolonged inactivity in a bed or wheelchair. Ironically, a common infection incurred in the hospital is C-DIF, an infection of the lower intestine that is actually caused by a combination of antibiotics taken by hospital patients. The C-DIF can become a serious condition that can linger for some time in the form of spores, and must be treated by a separate type of antibiotic.

There are two basic types of bacteria that can be treated by antibiotics. They are called gram-positive and gram-negative bacteria. Each causes certain types of bacterial infections and test differently when stained in a laboratory. Gram-positive bacteria tend to have a thicker cell wall. Like all bacteria, gram-positive and gram-negative varieties are living organisms that can be killed by antibiotics. Viruses are not living organisms and present different challenges in drug treatment procedures.

At the highest level, antibiotics can be classified as either bactericidal or bacteriostatic. Bactericidal drugs kill bacteria directly, while bacteriostatic drugs do not kill bacteria but prevent their growth. These classifications are based on laboratory behavior, and, in practice, both can be used to end a bacterial infection.

The most common broad classifications of antibiotics are aminoglycosides, carbaphenems, cephalopsorins, glycopeptides, macrolides, penicillins, polypeptides, qunilones, sulfonamides and tetracyclines. Each classification have their own targeted diseases, infections or types of complications.

The Solutions

Oral antibiotics are the most commonly used to treat infections and bacterial infectious diseases. In severe cases, antibiotics may be administered intravenously. In some cases, antibacterial ointments are used to treat skin conditions caused by bacteria.

Antibiotics are the most commonly sought after drugs from pharmaceutical companies. The development of a new and more powerful antibiotic can mean millions in income to the company which develops the drug. These drugs go through the same rigorous testing of any prescription drug and must indicate any possible resistance or side effects.

Many people have potentially deadly allergies to antibiotics, especially penicillin. If you are aware of these allergies, you must inform your Primary Care Physician and any specialist treating you to the presence of these allergies. The allergic reaction can cause death quickly, and, even when detected early, can leave a patient harmed permanently.

Food poisoning is caused by the introduction of a bacteria consumed by eating the item infected. Usually food poisoning is treated by bed rest and the use of fluids, with antibiotics not being necessary, in most cases, to treat the condition.

Modern doctors can choose from 100 different antibiotics to treat various types of infections and infectious diseases. The use of antibiotics by themselves or in combination usually depends on the nature of the disease or infection. Usually physicians will start with the most common antibiotic with the least likelihood of complications and move to other, more advanced, types of antibiotics. Here are a few common, newer antibiotics and what they are used to treat.

- Semisynthetic penicillin and vancomycin are used to treat the staphylococcal infections such as bactremia, with bacteria in the blood and characterized by high fever, chills, racing heart, pallor, agitation and joint pain.
- A topical treatment of mupirocin ointment will be used for the treatment of most skin infections. In severe cases, a patient may receive intravenous doses of advanced antibiotics such as oxacillin, methicillin and nafcillin.
- Penicillin and erythonycin are used to combat common forms of strep throat, infections of the threat caused by streptococcal bacteria. Untreated strep throat can lead to rheumatic fever or scarlet fever and must be treated promptly with antibiotics.
- Advanced antibiotics must be used to treat impetigo, a skin condition typified by lesions with itching and encrustment and lymphadenitis, red-streaked, painful lesions with fever, racing heart and lethargy.
- Penicillin and ampicillin are used to treat Group B streptococcal infections, usually infecting newborns and women above the age of 30 who have just given birth.
- Penicillin, amoxicillin and ampicillin are typically used to treat ottis media, fluid in the middle ear, and meningitis.
- Large doses of penicillin G, ampicillin, ceftriaxone or cefotaxime are used to treat the often dangerous condition of meningitis, found mostly in children under the age of five and those living in crowded conditions.
- Treatment for tetanus infections should begin within 72 hours and include the use of tetanus immune globulin or tetanus antitoxin for temporary infection followed by immunization treatment of tetanus toxoid.
- Oral doxycycline and tetracycline are usually used to treat lyme disease. This disease often is the result of the bite of an infected deer tick and can include skin lesions followed by a stiff neck, malaise, fatigue, chills, fever, headache, achiness and muscle pain. A stage two version of the disease can have severe cardiac and neurological symptoms. Other drugs used to treat lyme disease are penicillin, amoxicillin or cephalosporins.

Two emerging and growingly popular antibiotic treatments involve the use of bacteriophage therapy and enzybiotics. Bacteriophage therapy involves inserting viruses into bacteria and killing them from the inside. Enzybiotics, a new term, involves purifying the phage-encoded enzymes that kill the bacteria from within and using them as antibacterials from the outside.

The Resources

Visit the following Websites for more information on advances in antibiotics:

Family Doctor, *www.familydoctor.org*

Genome News Network, *www.genomenewsnetwork.org*

Discover Magazine, *www.discover.com*

Federal Drug Administration, *www.fda.gov*

HealthSquare, *www.healthsquare.com*

Phrma, *www.phrma.org*

Several books can be very helpful in explaining new antibiotic treatments such as:

Antibiotic Essentials, 2006 (Physicians Press, 2006)

Handbook of Antibiotics (Lippincott, Williams and Wilkins, 2000)

Antibiotics: Actions, Origins, Resistance (ASM Press, 2003)

Herbal Antibiotics (Newleaf, 2000)

The Antibiotic Paradox: How the Misuse of Antibiotics Destroys Their Curative Powers (Harper Collins, 2002)

Natural Alternatives to Antibiotics (Newleaf, 2003)

18

Understanding Psychotherapy

The Challenge

Mental illness not too long ago was seen as a failure by a patient to cope with normal life. The manifestations of mental illness which could be completely debilitating were misunderstood and, in some cases, resented by friends and family members who did not understand the nature of the condition. More and more mental illness is seen as just that, an illness that no one would bring on themselves. Mental illness can be diagnosed, but the process is much more difficult in many ways than diagnosing a physical condition. The process of treating and dealing with the mental illness can take a lot longer than treating a physical condition and may require a good therapist to adapt the treatment to the needs or changes of the patient. The challenge is when to recognize when one might be suffering from some form of mental illness, what type of specialist to visit to diagnose and deal with the illness, what types of treatment might be appropriate and evaluating when the treatment is working or not working. Dealing with a mental illness is never easy, but thanks to modern techniques, it can be accomplished and a person suffering from a mental illness does not have to face the possibility of being isolated from society, but work to reenter a mode of normal living with a healthy mental psyche.

The Facts

Psychotherapy covers a wide variety of conditions and disciplines but basically is an interspersonal, relational intervention to help patients cope with various problems of living. It generally means increasing an individual's sense of well being and reducing subjective discomforting experience. Psychotherapists use a variety of techniques that build relationships, increasing dialogue and communication and changing behavior to improve the mental health of a client or patient or to work on a group relationship such as a family.

There are three different types of psychotherapists you may consult depending on your condition:

- Counselors or social workers who may have a bachelor's degree and some experience in dealing with patients dealing with emotional difficulties;

- psychologists who usually have a PhD and are certified to practice in the state and
- psychiatrists who have an MD and can provide counseling services similar to what a counselor or psychologist offers, but can also prescribe drugs to treat the mental condition.

Most patient treatments follow what is called the medical model. This means identifying an illness and then providing a cure for it. For the most part, this is also the case when dealing with patients who are suffering mental disorders. But, not all psychotherapeutic approaches emphasize the medical model. Some practitioners believe they can be most effective by offering an educational or helper role. No matter what, a psychotherapist is expected and usually legally bound to do everything to respect patient confidentiality, thus building an essential feeling of trust between the therapist and the patient.

Unlike other forms of medical treatment, the most important part of psychotherapy is the relationship between the therapist and the patient and not the actual treatment. This therapeutic relationship has its own power to heal. Often, patients show improvement in behavior by just making an appointment for an initial session with a therapist.

Therapists have been using different techniques of treating children's mental illnesses for many years, but it has only been recently that therapists have recognized the particular needs of elder adults in dealing with mental illness. Often the illness may involve feelings of isolation, depression and anxiety. This type of psychotherapy has been called geropyschology. It used to be commonly thought that psychotherapy had little effect on the elderly, but this is increasingly being discarded through geropsychology. The therapy is often provided in a clinical setting and will combine the use of drugs with conversation. Geropsychologists recognize it may be more difficult to engage an elderly person into meaningful conversation and will work harder and within the most comfortable environments available to reach the patient and begin the healing process.

Managed care medical insurance will seldom reimburse you for more than 20 therapy sessions. The rest you will have to pay by yourself with an average fee of $100 per session. Also to acquire coverage, a therapist will usually have to discuss your case with a case manager who works for your insurance company and this sensitive information will be entered into a computer for future reference.

The Solutions

Conversation with a therapist is the usual method of engaging in psychotherapy and has shown excellent results since Sigmund Freud introduced the concept of psychoanalysis in the early 1900's. This conversation is designed to build a relationship, communicate and help the patient adopt behavior change strategies. Besides the spoken word, some counseling may involve using written words, artwork, drama, narrative story or therapeutic touch. However, within the conversation model and beyond that model are many types of psychotherapy techniques:

- Psychoanalysis, the earliest form of psychotherapy, uses conversation with patients to determine backgrounds, relationships and attitudes. Psychoanalysis usually looks at behaviors but can also work with feelings and thoughts.
- Group psychotherapy uses specific groups, especially family groups. The members of the group come to understand behaviors and how to change them based on their interactions and perceptions of earlier activities and feelings.
- Cognitive behavioral therapy is a type of psychotherapy primarily used to help with depression, anxiety disorders, phobias and other mental disorders. It recognizes distorted thinking and helps replace that with more realistic ideas and approaches to living.
- Expressive therapy uses artistic expression to treat clients. It uses creative arts such as movement, drama, art, music and writing. Expressive therapists believe treating a client through the expression of imagination in creative work can be very effective
- Drug therapy and electroshock therapy, in the correct cases, can help treat mental disorders. These therapies are usually administered by psychiatrists. The drugs help with depression and anxiety and often are used to treat a chemical imbalance in the patient that has caused the medical disorder.

Treating children with mental or development disorders can be particularly challenging and often means adapting forms of therapy used for adults. Most children under a certain age are not able to articulate their feelings as an adult might, so the therapist must use more artistic expressions, such as drawing, puppets, use of toys, to explore a child's perception of the world. Structured play, sometimes called theraplay, is often used to help children.

It is not unusual for a patient to experience very strong feelings toward the therapist. In destructive ways, these feelings can incorporate obsession, love or sexual attraction. These feelings can happen to anyone going through therapy, even if he or she is relatively happy with their existing relationships. This is often called transference. If not handled with skill, these feelings can be overpowering and allow the patient's other relationships to suffer. The patient may become extremely dependent upon their therapist and find they cannot perform simple life functions, such as making a purchase, without consulting the therapist.

Recognizing signs of a psychological disorder in yourself or others can be difficult. Often they are easiest to identify when seen as a natural progression. Because of sensitivity to a particular area or other's behavior, a person may adapt defensive signs of aggression or coldness that are not in the proper relationship to the stimulus. If left untreated, this type of defensiveness can develop into a full bloom of psychological symptoms such as depression, drug abuse, various anxieties, insomnias, personality disorders with signs of inappropriate behaviors and even violent aggression. Defenses are natural reactions to the stress of the world around us, but when the defense mechanisms fail, psychological symptoms can follow.

Finding a good therapist can be particularly challenging. You can consult a school counseling office or your company's Employment Assistance Program, but keep in mind, if a therapist does not appear on the recommended list, it may be because he or she is not included in the insurance program. Not all medical insurance obtained through the workplace will reimburse you for visits to therapist. Other methods of finding a good therapist are:

- Visiting a therapy center and applying for treatment at a less expensive rate;
- using trainees at therapy centers;
- checking the telephone book or online resources on finding a therapist;
- acting on the advice of your primary care physician;
- talking to friends and family who may have experience with a specific therapist and
- interviewing potential therapists to determine your rapport and their ability to communicate.

The Resources

Visit the following Websites for more information on psychotherapy:

The Clinical Psychologist, *www.bls.gov*

Department of Psychiatry, University of California, *www.psychiatry.ucsd.edu*

About Psychiatry, *www.aboutpsychotherapy.com*

Psychotherapy.net, *www.psychotherapy.net*

Mayo Clinic, *www.mayoclinic.com*

American Psychologists Association, *www.apa.org*

Division of Psychotherapy, *www.divisionofpsychotherapy.org*

Several books can be very helpful in learning about psychotherapy such as:

Doing Psychotherapy (Basic Books, 1980)

Mindfulness and Psychotherapy (The Guilford Press, 2005)

The Theory and Practice of Group Psychotherapy (Basic Books, 2005)

Current Psychotherapies (Wadsworth Publishing, 2007)

Attachment in Psychotherapy (The Guilford Press, 2007)

Ethics in Counseling and Psychotherapy: Standards, Research, and Emerging Issues (Wadsworth Publishing, 2005)

19

Physical Therapy Improvements

The Challenge

Once a medical procedure has been completed, or even in lieu of invasive treatments, a patient may undergo physical therapy. This type of therapy is used to complete a procedure and help a patient cope with an active lifestyle. Physical therapists have been more and more relied upon as an adjunct to medical treatment and physical therapists are now perceived as a vital part of a medical team. These therapists undergo rigorous training, and, in many cases see a patient more often and develop a close relationship. They are literally hands-on with the patient and their treatment goes far beyond simple body manipulation to deal with orthopedic issues, those that have been traditionally perceived as being the purview of a physical therapist. The challenge is for a patient to discuss the uses of physical therapy with a physician, develop a clear understanding of what a physical therapist can or cannot do, how to feel comfortable in the physical therapy, what is needed to maintain the physical therapy regimen away from a treatment center and how to analyze and communicate the positive or negative effects of the physical therapy.

The Facts

A physical therapist, especially in the case of beginning treatment without a physician referral, before treatment begins, must provide a patient in writing to alert the patient that the physical therapy may not be covered by the patient's health care insurance without a referral. This Notice of Advisory must, at the least, contain the following information:

- A statement of such advice and a statement attesting the patient has read the notice;
- the beginning date for treatment;
- the name and address of the patient;
- a patient signature and date on when the document was signed and
- a signature of the treating physical therapist and the date the physical therapist signed the form.

Physical therapy is the provision of services where movement and function are threatened by aging or injury. Physical therapy strives to restore full and functional movement to the body. The physical therapist's distinctive view of the body and its movement needs and potential is central to determining a diagnosis and strategy for intervention. The therapy will vary as to whether these settings will vary in relation to the condition. Physical therapy is concerned with maintaining health, prevention of debilitating conditions or rehabilitation of existing conditions.

Physical therapy used to be designed for the simple alleviation of pain caused by movement. Modern physical therapy techniques can now help with a variety of physical conditions and concerns.

- Back and neck pain;
- arthritis and other spinal and joint conditions;
- biomechanical issues and problems in muscular control;
- cerebral palsy and spinal bifida;
- heart and lung conditions including chronic obstructive pulmonary disease (COPD) and atelectasis (a partial or full collapse of the lung caused by blocked airways;
- headaches, both cervicogenic and tension type headaches;
- incontinence from stress factors and
- neurological conditions such as stroke and multiple sclerosis.

A physical therapist cannot just hang a sign up saying he or she is a physical therapist. Physical therapists are recognized health care professionals the same as physicians, nurses and technicians. Physical therapists must have a graduate degree from an accredited physical therapy program and pass a national licensing examination. Even though the minimum educational requirement to be a physical therapist is a master's degree, the therapist can seek and acquire a doctorate in physical therapy. A physical therapist must have a license in each state where he or she will practice.

You can get the most out of your physical therapy by understanding how the parts of your body most closely associated with physical therapy should properly perform. These include your knees, spine and primary ligaments.

A common type of condition meant to be alleviated by modern physical therapy is carpal tunnel syndrome. This condition is sometimes referred to as repetitive motion syndrome and is caused when the median nerve is compressed in the wrist. The syndrome is developed by constant use of the hands during keyboarding or manufacturing work. Carpal tunnel syndrome usually has a pins-and-needles sensation in the affected areas. The syndrome can be prevented by slightly elevating your keyboard and keeping your wrists straight and elbows at a 90-degree angle. It is also recommended to take frequent breaks from typing. You can help prevent carpal tunnel syndrome by stretching the tendons and ligaments with extension and flexing of the wrists.

The Solutions

You should understand how a physical therapist will approach your condition and what techniques are most commonly used in administering physical therapy. Physical therapy interventions normally include manual handling which uses electrotherapeutic and mechanical agents to enhance movement; functional training; providing various aids and appliances for use away from the physical therapy facility and communication of proper physical therapy techniques and the therapy's purpose in the recovery process. Intervention by use of physical therapy may also be used for prevention of impairments, enhancing the overall quality of life and general fitness in all ages and types of populations.

The first step in working with a physical therapist will be to go through a subjective examination, or interview, of your medical history and then proceeding to an objective examination of the specific physical condition based on the complaint. This process is designed to separate complaints based on serious pathology, to establish functional limitation, the diagnosis, guide the therapy choices and establish a baseline for monitoring progress.

Modern physical therapists have a variety of techniques available to them, the use of which depends on the condition and evaluation of the patient. These techniques are meant to be flexible and may vary based on changes in the patient's condition.

- Muscoloskeletal physical therapy use exercise prescription, manual therapy techniques such as joint mobilization and manipulation, soft tissue massage and various forms of electrophysical agents such as Cryotherapy, heat therapy, iontophoresis and electrotherapy.
- Cardiopulmonary physical therapy is designed to treat acute problems such as asthma, chest infections and trauma, as well as the preparation and recovery of patients from major surgery. The therapy is used for all ages of patients.
- Neurological physical therapy is treatment of neurological conditions and uses exercises to restore motor functions. One of the newer techniques in this type of therapy is the use of movement science frameworks.
- Integumentary physical therapy treats conditions of the skin and related organs including wounds and burns. Treatment interventions include wounds and burns debridement, the use of dressings, and scar prevention and reduction.

Under the supervision and the treatment plan of a licensed physical therapist you may receive treatment from a physical therapist assistant. The assistant is also a licensed health care professional and has completed an approved four-to-six year college program in physical therapy. They must also pass a written licensure examination.

A physical therapist nowadays may practice in a variety of settings, each offering advantages and disadvantages to the convenience of the patient. These settings include hospitals, clinics, private practices, care at home, schools and in the workplace. The facility should be physically accessible with handicapped parking, curb cuts, ramps and disabled restrooms and should have a Telecommunications Device for the Deaf (TED). Be sure to explore the possibility that the physical therapy practice includes house visits.

You should constantly be evaluating the performance of your physical therapist by asking the following questions:

- Has a licensed physical therapist performed your evaluation?
- Has the physical therapist thoroughly involved you in developing goals and an individualized treatment plan?
- Was your privacy properly maintained?

Many conditions leading to physical therapy are caused by falls in the house. These can be prevented in a variety of ways.

- Clean up spills soon after they occur.
- Remove all small throw rugs.
- Install rails in the bathtub or shower.
- Remove clutter from all stairways?

The Resources

Visit the following Websites for more information on physical therapy treatments:

American Physical Therapy Association, *www.apta.org*

Journal of Physical Therapy, *www.ptjournal.org*

Physical Therapist.com, *www.physicaltherapist.com*

International Association of Healthcare Practitioners, *www.iahp.com*

Mindful Movement and Physical Therapy, *www.mindfulmovement.biz*

New York State Office of Education, *www.op.nysed.gov*

Several books can be very helpful in explaining physical therapy training, evaluation and treatments such as:

The American Physical Therapy Association Book of Body Maintenance and Repair (Owl Books, 1999)

Orthopedic Physical Therapy Secrets (Hanley & Belfus, 2006)

Physical Therapy for Children (Saunders, 2005)

Starting and Managing Your Own Physical Therapy Practice (Jones and Bartlett Publishers, Inc., 2004)

Introduction to Physical Therapy (Mosby, 2006)

Physical Therapy Ethics (F.A. Davis Company, 2003)

20

Improvements in Treating Hip Conditions

The Challenge

Of the major orthopedic conditions that can cause pain and debilitation are hip problems. These problems can be caused by work, play or simply heredity. The symptoms can include terrific pain that will affect you in almost every aspect of your life. Unlike in the past, when hip conditions were treated with primitive orthopedic devices, modern treatment methods for hip conditions can use a variety of medications and surgery to relieve the condition and restore the patient to a normal existence. The challenge is to recognize the difference between fleeting pain caused by a temporary usage vs. hip pain that indicates a much more chronic condition, having that condition adequately diagnosed and then progressing through a series of treatments to alieve the condition. Hip problems do not have to limit your lifestyle and with the proper attention and approach, can be conquered and allow you to live a pain-free life.

The Facts

Hip pain and a deteriorating hip joint can be caused and exacerbated by a variety of causes:

- Arthritis or bursitis, debilitating conditions, that cause gradual swelling or deterioration of joint tissue can cause enough pain to constitute a major hip problem;
- a childhood injury to the hip, typically playing sports, that can cause the hip to deteriorate with pain and loss of movement and
- adult injuries playing sports or doing heavy work that can have a long-term effect on the hip.

The two most important physicians in the diagnosis, short-term and long-term, in hip condition treatment are your orthopedic surgeons and your physical therapist. You primary care physician will usually refer you to a therapist. The therapist will test your mobility and the pain involved and use x-rays or other imaging tools to take a look at your hip. In some cases, they may use an arthroscope to get into the joint area and see what your condition looks like visually. The orthopedic surgeon, whether they use surgery or less invasive techniques, will probably want you to work with a physical therapist. Under the right conditions, a physical therapist may be able to help you regain hip motion and lower your pain through a series of exercises and stretches. If surgery is done on your hip, including a hip replacement, a physical therapist will be vital in guiding your recovery and helping you regain as much movement as possible.

According to the American Academy of Orthopedic Surgeons, AAOS, there will be a boom in hip treatments because of the natural aging of the population. More and more baby boomers will be entering their sixties and may want to maintain a certain level of participation in sports and exercise. This is prompting orthopedic surgeons to use advanced methods of detection, evaluation, treatment and surgical and non-surgical options for musculoskeletal conditions of the hips and other joints. Age is not always a determinant of hip problems. Younger people, even those in their 20's, may be more susceptible to hip injury due to increased activity than previous generations.

A rapid replacement for x-rays that is more accurate and will not deliver radiation to the patient is the use of gadolinium-arthrogram magnetic resonance imaging, MRI. In this procedure, contrast material is injected into the hip joint, allowing for specific views and sequencing. The images on damaged or torn cartilage, cartilage loss or loose bodies within the hip do not normally appear on x-rays, conventional magnetic resonance imaging or computerized tomography, CT, scans.

If the extent of the hip condition has deteriorated to a certain point, orthopedic surgeons will probably want to do a total hip replacement. This used to involve using a ball and socket that could cause the patient as much pain as the hip problem. Modern hip replacement removes the affected hip joint and replaces it with a custom-fitted appliance that will recreate the movement of the hip. Metal-on-metal replacements and ceramic replacements both have the same level of deterioration after they are placed.

One of the more common hip problems among children is hip dysplasia. Hip dysplasia is a congenital condition where there is a problem with the formation of the hip joint or the location. There are many possible causes of hip dysplasia, which can be very painful. Depending on the age of the patient, hip dysplasia may be treated with a brace, harness or surgery.

Other conditions that can affect the hip besides arthritis are hip bursitis and tendonitis. Bursitis can be caused by athletic activity, injuries or post-surgical complications. Tendonitis is where the hip tendons become inflamed because of overuse of the joint. Tendonitis can be brought on by the sudden implementation of an exercise program after relative inactivity.

The Solutions

Many patients suffering from hip or other orthopedic conditions are content for many years in using pain medication to help them lead a normal life. But, pain medication is just a stopgap and will not cure the problem. Eventually the pain medication will lose its effectiveness and the physician and patient will have to make tough decisions on whether to up the dosage or strength of the pain medication or looking at a more permanent solution that will eliminate the pain. The danger in dealing with increasingly large doses of pain medication is the possibility of causing a chemical dependency or addiction to the pain killer.

Another chemical alternative to hip surgery is to use cortisone injections, delivered directly to the affected joint. The cortisone, a form of steroid, can effectively reduce painful swelling of the joint tissue and tissue surrounding the joint but can carry potentially dangerous side effects to the patient. Like pain medication, the patient may reach the point where the medication is not as effective and has to be used more.

Some patients experiencing hip problems may gave less invasive treatment. These treatments include less invasive hip arthroplasty, or joint replacement and hip resurfacing that treats the hip joint without removal of the actual joint. Hip arthroscopy is a biologic alternative to total hip replacement and uses an instrument to smooth out the hip, repair a cartilage tear or remove a loose body. Physicians must decide whether the additional risks of these less-invasive techniques are worth the benefits and know that not all patients are candidates for these types of surgery. This will depend on the type of injury and the patient's overall health.

Hip resurfacing is often recommended for younger patients who may face the prospect of needing a total hip replacement. The resurfacing is called for because hip replacements only have a certain life span, which varies widely from one patient to another depending on the condition and level of activity. An older patient may never have to worry about receiving a second replacement in his or her lifetime, but this added replacement may become necessary for a younger patient. This makes the use of resurfacing more desirable for a younger patient.

It is important to stay active during recovery from a hip replacement and follow the specific requirements of the physical therapist. A patient receiving a hip replacement will not see significant improvement if the joint is not regularly exercised. Those who recover from hip replacement can remain physically active as long as they adhere to restrictions recommended by their orthopedic surgeon or physical therapist.

The Resources

Visit the following Websites for more information on hip treatment and replacements:

American Academy of Orthopedic Surgeons, *www.aaos.org/news*

About Orthopedics, *www.about.com*

Bandolier, *www.jr2.ox.ac.uk/bandolier*

EMedicine Journal, *www.emedicine.com/orthopedics*

Johns Hopkins Department of Orthopedic Surgery, *www.hopkinsmedicine.org*

The Internet Journal of Orthopedic Surgery, *www.ispub.com*

American Board of Orthopedic Surgery, *www.abos.org*

Several books can be very helpful in learning about hip treatment and replacements such as:

Early Hip Disorders: Advances in Detection and Minimally Invasive Treatment (Springer, 2003)

Heal Your Hips: How to Prevent Hip Surgery—and What to Do If You Need It (Wiley, 1999)

Clinical Challenges in Orthopedics: The Hip (Informa Healthcare, 2001)

Current Diagnosis & Treatment in Orthopedics (McGraw-Hill/Appleton & Lange, 2000)

Getting Hip: Recovery from A Total Hip Replacement (AuthorHouse, 2004)

Your Complete Guide to Total Hip Replacements: Before, During, And After Surgery (Idyll Arbor, 2004)

21

Improvements in Treating Knee Conditions

The Challenge

Very few joints in the human body experience the same possibility of injury and disease as the knees. The knees are the shock absorbers for the weight of the body and are used in almost every type of physical activities. The extent of this use means the knees can be affected by behavioral and other conditions to cause loss of movement and substantial pain. From weekend warrior to professional athletes, knee injuries are debilitating and can take much time and effort to correct. These corrections may mean the use of prescription drugs, minimally invasive surgical techniques or major surgery to correct a problem. Recovering from a knee injury can mean weeks or months of therapy. Drug treatments may last a lifetime and carry their own issues in terms of side effects and the benefits of the drugs. The challenge is to recognize what types of behavior may cause knee injuries, what are involved in chronic knee conditions that do not involve injury, deciding on a regimen of treatment and then changing lifestyles to ease the possibility of the knee condition continuing or returning. With the proper and informed approach to knee conditions and understanding what is new in treating them, you can help alleviate the pain and lack of mobility from most knee conditions and begin to live a more normal lifestyle with a minimum of discomfort.

The Facts

The knee joint is made of three bones: the femur, the tibia and the patella. The proximal tibia-fibula joint is also in the knee but is not injured very often. The joint surface is covered by articulate cartilage which provides a smooth, lubricated gliding surface for proper knee motion. Proper function of the knee depends primarily on intact ligaments. This include the anterior cruciate ligament, ACL; the posterior cruciate ligament, PCL, the medical collateral ligament, MCL; and the lateral collateral ligament, LCL. The medial and lateral menisci are located within the joint between the femur and tibia. The menisci work as shock absorbers in the knee. The front of the knee is protected by the patella or kneecap. The knee is controlled by quadriceps muscles and the hamstrings.

Based on the makeup of the knee joint, there are several conditions that may be caused in the most common injuries to the knee.

- Patella tendonitis is a common injury caused by overuse or repetitive trauma to the extensor mechanism, often while playing basketball or volleyball. Symptoms of patella tendonitis are pain in the front of the knee over the patella tendon. Treatment usually involves a period of rest for the knee followed by modifications in activity that are designed to limit the high activity of sports. Stretching and strengthening exercises are also frequently prescribed. The quadriceps tendon may also become sore in a similar fashion and includes tenderness in the soft tissue just above the patella. Treatment is basically the same as an injury to the patella tendon.

- Bursitis affects the bursae, synovial lined cavities that cover the bony prominence around the knee. Repetitive trauma from activity and overuse results in chronic irritation of the bursae and includes fluid collection. Housemaid's knee is an inflammation of the prepatellar bursa. Treatment for bursitis is directed at the elimination of the irritating activity and the application of ice. A comprehensive knee wrap is also sometimes helpful to treat bursitis. In some extreme cases, fluid is drained from the bursa.

- Patellofemoral pain and chondromalacia patella is pain in the front of the knee and is a common complaint caused by patella malalignment, fractures, synovial plica, bursitis, tendonitis and patella instability. The initial treatment for these conditions is usually non-operative, but, depending on the condition's response, some type of surgery may be needed. Softening and erosive changes to the surface of the patella are called chondromalacia. This condition is treated by modifying activity and ice. Later, an exercise program may be initiated focusing on strength and stretching.

- Anterior cruciate ligament, ACL, injuries are the most debilitating to athletes and used to mean the end of a career. The injury is almost always caused by playing competitive sports. The planting of the foot and knee twists with a change of direction usually cause the injury. Physical examination, x-rays and MRI scanning are used to detect a ACL injury. Treatment may be non-operative and involve a program of physical therapy to restore motion and strength. Reconstructive surgery almost always uses an arthroscopic approach, followed by a rehabilitation program. Well-trained athletes may take six to eight weeks to regain movement in the ACL following non-operative therapy and six to nine months after surgery.

- Posterior cruciate ligament, PCL, injuries are less common than ACL injuries. They are usually caused by a fall on a hyper flexed knee, such as an injury caused by impacting a dashboard during an accident. Treatment can be non-operative or operative depending on the extent of the injury.

- Menisci tears usually are caused by a twisting injury. The medial meniscus is the one usually torn. MRIs have been shown to be useful in determining meniscal tears. Some meniscal tears may heal with simple rest and behavior modification, but often the surgeon will need to use operative treatment. This is usually done with an arthroscope, followed by an exercise program to restore motion and strength.

- Knee arthritis, also called osteoarthritis, usually affects patients over the age of 50. This is a progressive disease that eats away at the cartilage of the joint. Treating knee arthritis usually starts with non-operative drug therapies, such as cortisone and, in some cases, may progress to surgery. Occasionally ultrasound can work to treat knee arthritis.

The Solutions

Often times lifestyle will cause injuries to the knee that could have been avoided. The most common of lifestyle influences on knee health are weight and exercise, including playing sports. Those who are overweight put tremendous pressure on the knee joints, and this pressure can cause serious injuries that are difficult to treat. Exercise and playing sports that depend on rapid starts and stops as well as twisting of the lower trunk can also cause knee injuries. The best way to treat these type of knee injuries is to lose weight and be careful during exercise or sports. Wrapping the knee with a flexible brace can also help avoid common knee problems from activity.

There are two types of common surgery used to repair knee injuries. Full knee surgery, usually resulting in a knee replacement, may be recommended for severe knee injury. More and more orthopedic surgeons are using arthroscopic surgery where a tube with a cutting device is inserted into the knee. This arthroscope allows surgeons to see the nature of the injury and repair it without having to do major surgery. The recovery from arthroscopic surgery to the knee usually takes less time than full surgery and involves less discomfort for the patient.

Besides losing weight and modifying activity, surgeons may recommend a program that builds up the strength in the thigh muscles. Strengthening these muscles can help reduce the pressure put on the knee.

Common medications for the treatment of knee conditions include anti-inflammatories and steroids. These are designed to reduce swelling in the knee and restore pain-free motion. Sometimes with operations on the knee, a physician may prescribe painkillers to help with post-operative discomfort.

Other, newer drug treatments for injuries of the knee have moved beyond anti-inflammatory drugs and cortisone treatments. Orthopedic surgeons are now using hyaluronic acid, a thick fluid that is removed from healthy joints and injected into the injured knee. Most experts do not know how hyaluronic acid works, which until 1997 was used to treat race horses, but it can help alleviate knee pain and reduce inflammation for up to six months. Topical painkillers, ointments applied directly to the knee, may help reduce the pain of osteoarthritis. The cream most commonly used is called Celadin and may show soothing effects within 30 minutes of application. The FDA has approved the use of over-the-counter capsacin, sold under a variety of brand names, for temporary relief of arthritis pain in the knee.

The Resources

Visit the following Websites for more information on treating knee conditions:

The Knee Society, *www.kneesociety.org*

University of Michigan, *www.med.umich.edu*

Wrong Diagnosis, *www.wrongdiagnosis.com*

Orthopedics About, *www.orthopedics.about.com*

Arthritis Treatment and Relief, *www.arthritis-treatment-and-relief.com*

Mayo Clinic, *www.mayoclinic.com/health/knee-pain*

Carticel, *www.carticel.com*

Several books can be very helpful in learning about treating knee conditions such as:

Yoga for Healthy Knees: What You Need to Know for Pain Prevention and Rehabilitation (Rodmell Press, 2005)

The Knee Crisis Handbook: Understanding Pain, Preventing Trauma, Recovering from Knee Injury and Building Healthy Knees for Life (Rodale Books, 2003)

What Your Doctor May Not Tell You About Knee Pain and Surgery: Learn the Truth About MRIs and Common Misdiagnoses—And Avoid Unnecessary Surgery (Warner Books, 2002)

A Patient's Guide to Knee and Hip Replacement: Everything You Need to Know (Fireside, 1999)

Heal Your Knees: How to Prevent Knee Surgery and What to Do If You Need It (M. Evans and Company, 2004)

Total Knee Replacement and Rehabilitation: The Knee Owner's Manual (Hunter House, 2004)

22

Improvements in Treating Back Conditions

The Challenge

There are few medical conditions that are as painful and potentially debilitating as suffering from chronic back pain. With a back condition you may experience pain doing basic movements, even walking, sitting down or lying down. Sometimes it can feel like there is little or nothing you can do to relieve the pain except rely on pain killers that can have side effects beyond their ability to ease the pain. A back condition may be experienced at a later stage in life, but younger people are not immune to the effects of a back condition either from exercise, normal activity or congenital conditions. There are some common treatment options, such as surgery, you can investigate to relieve the pain of a back condition, but it may be just as worthwhile to explore other treatment options that do not involve radical forms of treatment that may require lengthy therapy and may not have any guarantees of permanently solving the condition. An old statement is that once you have a back condition, you always will, but the condition does not have to radically alter your quality of life. The challenge is to recognize what types of behavior may lead to back conditions and how to avoid them, how to recognize a chronic back condition from simple, temporary pain and what treatment options are available to you. Using the proper decisions can help you conquer the effects of back pain and lead a normal lifestyle.

The Facts

Developing a chronic back problem may not be associated with one action, but is a condition developed over time and in ways that are not noticeable until they are causing you pain. There are certain actions that can bring on or aggravate back conditions:

- Lack of exercise;
- beginning an exercise program that is more of a shock to the back than it is beneficial;
- poor posture;
- being generally out of shape and overweight, especially if you have developed a large stomach;

- an accident involving a fall and
- poor lifting practices that can put undue strain on the back.

If you develop potential back conditions you should start with an initial assessment from your primary care physician. You must be detailed in the effects of the back condition, particularly if the pain is traveling to other areas of your body. Your primary care physician will then likely refer you to an orthopedic surgeon who will help develop a treatment regimen for your back. One of the last elements to be considered would be some type of back surgery, because of the traumatic effect of the surgery and the uncertainty of the surgery success. Finally, you would be referred to a qualified and professional physical therapist who can further help develop an exercise program and work with you on a regular basis to make sure you are following the routine properly and monitoring how this routine is benefiting your back condition. Your physician and therapist should be willing to alter the regimen to try to continue to alieve the condition and not have what is being done to you written in stone.

Keeping your body active is key to avoiding back problems. If you allow your muscles, bones and tendons to fall into disuse, they will start to give you pain, especially in a area as susceptible to chronic pain as your back. You must attempt to stay as active as possible, keeping in mind other conditions that can affect your ability to move. You should rely on gentle exercise that will slowly build strong back and stomach muscles. These muscles will help support your spine and promote flexibility. Walking or cycling can be easy to incorporate into your lifestyle and will help build strength in your back. Swimming can be a particularly effective form of back exercise because the water helps provide support for your body, although you should consult an exercise expert since some strokes may not be good for you.

Bringing your weight down can be very helpful in reducing back pain. Explore doing an aerobic exercise that can help you lose weight and maintain a healthy diet that is high in fruits, grains and vegetables rather than meat and fat. A poor diet can go beyond not maintaining your weight, but can actually contribute to making your back weaker and more susceptible to injury.

In many cases, back pain can be temporary and transient and may require bed rest or simple pain killers. However there are some conditions that, if they manifest themselves with back pain, should bring you immediately to your physician.

- Severe back pain that does not quickly subside;
- radiating pain from your back to your legs;
- bowel or bladder incontinence;
- leg weakness;
- persistent fever and
- color changes in the legs or feet.

The Solutions

Be sure to consult with your doctor or physical therapist before beginning a regular routine of exercises to heal your back. They can help you determine which types of exercise are the safest. Your doctor should be able to give you a personal assessment based on the nature of your back condition and on other aspects of your overall physical health.

If you do go to an exercise class to strengthen your back, make sure the class is run by a qualified teacher and that the teacher is aware you have a bad back. Many commonly performed exercises may not be appropriate for you because of your back condition. To avoid bad effects from your new exercise, here are some suggestions for getting started.

- Choose exercises that are suitable for your level, if you are just beginning a back exercise program, start gradually and work your way up.
- Always take the exercise at your own pace and do not feel you have to keep up with the rest of the class.
- Drink plenty of water before, during and after your exercise session.
- Make sure you do gentle warm-up stretches both before and after your exercise session.
- Wear comfortable, supportive footwear and comfortable clothing that allows your body to move easily.
- Enjoy yourself during the exercise. Keeping a good mental attitude will maintain your motivation to continue your exercise program. Get to know the other people in your class and enjoy their company as part of a social situation.
- Cease any exercise activity if it causes your back to hurt and consult with your exercise teacher on an alternative to this type of activity.
- Do not eat a large or heavy meal before exercising.
- Do not perform fitness or aerobic exercises on a hard stone or concrete floor. Perform these exercises on wood floors with some give or on carpeting that helps cushion the shock to your system from the exercise.
- Avoid exercising during a period if you feel ill.
- Be aware of how the exercise you are doing will put weight or excessive strain on your back, aggravating rather than alleviating the condition.

Posture is an important element of maintaining back health. There are several aspects to proper posture. When standing, try to avoid rounding your back, hunching your shoulders and tensing your neck if you feel stressed. When sitting use an upright chair for support of your lower back, use a small cushion or rolled-up towel to support the small of your back and get up and stretch every 20 to 30 minutes. When moving and lifting, look at alternatives such as pushing or pulling an object, do not lift objects that are too heavy for you, bend your knees and keep your back straight with your feet apart, do not lift and twist at the same time, lift and carry close to your body and bend your knees rather than your back when putting a load down.

There are a variety of treatments frequently recommended to alleviate back pain.

- Heat therapy for back spasms or similar conditions;
- medications such as muscle relaxants, narcotics, non-steroidal and anti-inflammatory drugs;
- exercise programs;
- massage therapy from an experienced practitioner;
- manipulation provided by a chiropractor, osteopath or physical therapist;
- acupuncture;
- cortisone treatments to reduce swelling;
- surgery including discectomy surgery, spinal fusion, artificial disc replacement, kyphoplasty or vertebroplasty and spinal cord stimulation.

The Resources

Visit the following Websites for more information on understanding and treating back conditions:

BBC Co., *www.bbc.co.uk*

Low Back Pain Facts, *www.ninds.nih.gov/disorders/backpain*

Patient Information Medical Journal, *www.spine-health.com*

Alternative Back Pain Health Advice, *www.acumedic.com*

Spine Universe, *www.spineuniverse.com*

Health A to Z, *www.healthatoz.com*

National Center for Complementary and Alternative Medicine, *www.nccam.nih.gov*

Several books can be very helpful in learning about understanding and treating back conditions such as:

Ageless Spine, Lasting Health: The Open Secret to Pain-Free Living and Comfortable Aging (Synergy Books, 2006)

Back Stability (Human Kinetics Publishing, 2000)

Back Pain Solutions: How to Help Yourself with Poster-Movement Therapy and Education (Extensional Pub, 2001)

Back in Control: Your Complete Prescription for Preventing, Treating and Eliminating Back Pain from Your Life (M. Evans and Company, 2003)

Rapid Recovery from Back and Neck Pain: A Nine-Step Recovery Plan (Health Advisory Group, 2002)

Backache Survival: The Holistic Medical Treatment Program for Chronic Low Back Pain (Tarcher, 2003)

23

Improvements in Treating Eye Conditions

The Challenge

Nothing can be more frightening than developing a debilitating eye condition that can lead to a radical reduction in sight or perhaps even blindness. Unless we have dealt with being blind from birth or an early age, the prospect of adapting to an eye condition that can lead to loss in slight is daunting to say the least. How will we cope with the lack of eyesight? Will our driving and ability to get around be curtailed? Is the treatment proposed really going to work, or simply provide an avenue to discomfort and frustration. Luckily, like many areas of medicine, treatment of most eye conditions has improved remarkably over the last few decades with non-invasive treatments such as eye exercises, medications and laser surgery replacing older techniques that could possibly do as much harm as good. While no one wants to deal with the implications of an eye condition, it is possible more and more to successfully treat the conditions and allow patients to lead normal lives. The challenge is to understand the nature of the most common forms of eye conditions, not all of which depend on the age of the patient or injury, identify which type of eye professional can best work with you, how to select from several possible treatments and how to follow-up on any eye treatments to maximize recovery and reduce the time involved to return to basic living. You can effectively fight eye conditions with the right help, you simply have to provide some understanding and flexibility in the diagnoses and treatments.

The Facts

Often medical science does not know why a specific eye condition arises in one person, but not another. They simply must deal with the condition as they find it and understand its treatment. However, there are several factors that may contribute to eye problems that vary widely in their severity:

- Eye strain in misusing computers or not maintaining an updated prescription for eye glasses can be troublesome and lead to a temporary loss in sight.
- Work issues such as working in poor lighting or performing work in a dusty environment without proper eye protection, such as simple industrial goggles, can lead to eye conditions from absorbing construction dust.

- Accidents that have objects penetrate the eyes or the tissues around the eyes are unpredictable and capable of causing great damage.
- Congenital conditions such as glaucoma can be inherited from other close family members.
- The effects of diseases, such as diabetes, can have a debilitating effect on the eye which has to be treated specially as a side effect of a larger disease.

One of the most common eye problems encountered by patients is glaucoma. Glaucoma is caused by elevated pressure in the eye. This is due to an imbalance in pressure in the aqueous that fills the eye. It depends on a delicate balance between production and drainage and determines the eyes' intraocular pressure. In glaucoma, the outflow of fluid becomes blocked. If left untreated, the high pressure can damage the optic nerve and retina of the eye. Medical treatments start with simple eye drops to help lower the pressure. The body has a limit for how little aqueous fluid is inside the eye and this can be a problem with treating glaucoma with drugs. Surgery such as trabeculectomy is a common type of glaucoma surgery that involves making a tiny filtering valve in the sclera, or white of the eye. New developments in treating glaucoma has led to the use of a procedure called viscocanalostomy, which involves removing an internal layer of scleral tissue, opening a new pathway for fluid to drain.

Another common eye condition is macular degeneration. It is the most common cause of vision loss in people over 50. It effects the retina and is caused by hardening of the arteries that nourish the retina. Signs of macular degeneration include loss of central vision, difficulty reading or performing tasks that need the ability to see in detail and distorted vision. Photodynamic therapy can help with macular degeneration but is not a cure-all. Nutrition and lifestyle changes are also recommended for treating macular degeneration.

Cataracts are a natural clouding of the lens by fluid within the eye. They are the leading cause of vision loss for adults 55 and older. Cataracts can be corrected through surgery, but often are a condition that simply has to be adapted to.

The Solutions

It is imperative you visit an eye physician as soon as possible if you believe you have developed eye conditions that are new and unexpected. The sooner the physician is able to do a diagnosis and begin some form of treatment, the better are your chances in combating the condition. If you wear eyeglasses or contact lenses, you should be visiting for a basic eye examination on a yearly basis to make sure no other conditions have arisen or your sight is not degenerating beyond what is considered normal parameters. At the very least these visits may lead to upgraded prescriptions for your eyeglasses, at the most they will lead to a reference to another eye professional who can evaluate your specific condition.

It is important, as part of the care of your eye, to know which type of eye professional physician may be available to you and what each can offer in terms of specialization.

These professionals in eye care traditionally include:

- An ophthalmologist is a medical doctor whose training includes a bachelor degree, four years of medical school, a one year internship and three to four year residency program. Ophthalmologists are trained to diagnose and treat eye diseases and conditions with primarily medications and surgery. Some will specialize in eye diseases such as glaucoma.
- An optometrist has a bachelor's degree and has completed four years of additional education at an accredited optometry school. Optometrists specialize in prescribing and fitting glasses and are usually part of the staff of an eyeglass center. They can also detect early stages of eye diseases. Your optometrist may work closely with your ophthalmologist to diagnose and treat more serious eye conditions.
- An ocularist is specially trained to fit prosthetic eyes in place after a catastrophic accident or to help cover eye disfigurements. Ocularists must complete a five year apprentice program and pass a board examination for proper certification.
- Orthoptists specialize in evaluating the visual system and muscle function, especially with infants, children or younger people. They will work along with optometrists and ophthalmologists to provide non-surgical treatments to correct muscle imbalances and associated eye problems. Orthopists must complete two years of specialized training as well as a board examination.
- An optician is specially trained to make and fit eyeglasses and contact lenses. They require two years of training prior to taking a board examination.
- Ophthalmic medical personnel will assist the physician in the diagnoses of eye conditions, the treatment of the disease or injury and the after-care of the patient. The Joint Commission on Allied Health Personnel offers certification on three different levels: certified ophthalmic assistant, certified ophthalmic technician and certified ophthalmic medical technologist. Each level of certification requires specific education, skills and experience over the previous level.
- Certified ophthalmic retinal photographers specialize in photography of the eye that will be used for diagnosis and documentation of eye conditions. These professionals may become certified after sitting for a board examination and passing a skill evaluation.
- An ophthalmic registered nurse has received specialized training in eye care and certification which goes beyond the two to four years of normal nursing education.

One of the most highly-praised and used methods to improve eyesight and mostly eliminate the need for eyeglasses is through LASIK surgery. LASIK stands for laser assisted in situ keratomileusis. The LASIK improves vision by reshaping the cornea. The procedure is simple, relatively non-invasive and can be performed in a physician's office. The laser is used to open a flap in the retina, allowing the physician to realign the underlying tissues. Patients can see an almost instantaneous improvement in vision after LASIK and will need to use eye drops for about a week to promote healing.

Maintaining eye exams is important for an adult, but it is vital for children. This is because vision parameters can be set by the age of 11 and often eye problems are not reported by the child because he or she can quickly adapt to them. You should look out for these obvious symptoms:

- Eye alignment;
- winking, closing one eye while reading or watching television;
- rubbing, blinking and squeezing;
- watery, crusty or red-rimmed eyes;
- white pupils or other unnatural colors and
- complaints of headaches.

Although consulting with an eye physician is always recommended, there are several methods a patient can employ to deal with eye conditions that do not depend on a physician's care. These include avoiding prolonged use of the eyes, non-prescription eyedrops that can help deal with dry eyes, itching and redness often due to environmental factors and avoiding bacteria contact. Stay away from standard home remedies such as flushing the eyes with boric acid.

The Resources

Visit the following Websites for more information on eye conditions:

St. Luke's Eyecare Center, *www.stlukeseye.com/news*

American Board of Opticianry, *www.abo.ncle.org*

All About Vision, *www.allaboutvision.com*

Medscape, *www.medscape.com*

Kids Health, *www.kidshealth.org*

American Academy of Ophthalmology, *www.aao.org*

Vision Channel, *www.visionchannel.net*

Several books can be very helpful in learning about eye conditions such as:

Prevention and Treatment of Some Common Eye Conditions (E. Michael Geiger, 2002)

Microcurrent Stimulation: Miracle Eye Cure? (North Atlantic Books, 2001)

Refractive Eye Surgery A Consumer's Complete Guide: LASIK, IntraLASIK, Epi-LASIK, CK, Implantable Contact Lenses and other Surgical Eye Procedures (BookSurge Publishing, 2006)

Healing the Eye the Natural Way: Alternate Medicine and Macular Degeneration (North Atlantic Books, 2001)

All About Your Eyes (Duke University Press, 2006)

Common Eye Diseases and their Management (Springer, 2005)

24

Drug Treatments in Combination

The Challenge

Taking prescriptions can be a challenge for a variety of reasons. You need to know what you are being prescribed and why, the expectations of the treatment and what side effects to expect from the prescription. You need clear instructions on when to take the prescription and what type of food or drink, both regular and alcoholic, that can be taken with the medication. Another aspect of taking prescriptions that will be important to your treatment and overall health is how the new prescription may interact with what you are already taking. This interaction can have profound effects on how your treatment is progressing in its healing and how your overall health might be affected. These effects have the potential to make you feel sicker than you already do, even though the new prescription is doing what it is supposed to do. The effects may deter you from taking the new prescription or lead you to self-medicate in a sense by determining how to combine the new prescription with the old. The challenge is to recognize what the likelihood is for debilitating effects from combining new prescriptions with the ones you are already taking, how the new prescription should be properly taken, detecting when the new prescription either is not having the desired effect or not combining well with what you are already taking and how to communicate your concerns over prescription effect and combination are with your physician. When handled properly, and in an informed manner, prescriptions can do miraculous things to treat your condition, when mishandled they can cause as much harm as good. When you know the difference, you will be better able to work to treat your condition.

The Facts

Often drug treatments are designed to include one or more different types of prescriptions that are designed to act in combination to work on your condition. These drug combinations are especially used in treating long-term conditions such as HIV/AIDS, diabetes or hypertension. More often the drug combinations are not planned ahead of time, but are recognized as part of treatment for another condition that has very little or no relationship to an existing condition. It is quite often that this type of drug combination can cause you the most problems.

The Annals of Internal Medicine are an excellent and unbiased method to determining the history of prescriptions, their effects and their interaction. Almost every prescription drug will be covered by an article or study by the Annals of Internal Medicine and new prescriptions are usually explained by the Annals soon after the prescription is made available. Annals can help patients better understand the complicated or often mystifying language of modern medicine. The main information aspects of the Annals are the Summaries for Patients which were presented for information only. They are not a summary for the information that will be provided by your physician. Contact your physician with any questions from the information in the Annals' Summaries. The Summaries can be reproduced for not-for-profit purposes only and not be used by physicians, organizations or pharmaceutical companies to help sell the prescription and generate income from it.

Sometimes a drug combination can be used to help fight nausea, other digestive concerns or hypertension caused by the original prescription. These other prescriptions may not be used to fight the actual condition but as a palliative to treat other conditions. The danger is to load up with a variety of drugs to not only go after the condition but treat the reaction of the prescription. The result can be a spiral of chasing one type of prescription with another to the ill effect to the patient.

Physicians are usually very careful in combining drugs, but may use their desire to treat a condition by combining drugs in the real hopes of effectively treating or even curing the condition. This desire can occasionally mean using drug prescription combinations that can cause difficulties. Every so often a physician may be tempted to experiment with your treatment by using their own guesswork and experience in the prescription of drugs. This is rare, but not unknown. The key is to know when you are properly being prescribed and not being used as a guinea pig.

The Solutions

There are two medical professionals that can help you with determining the nature of your drug combinations and how that may affect you. One is your physician who can answer your questions about what to expect from a new prescription and give you a general idea of what to be aware of in combining the new prescription with what you are already taking. Another important part of your medical team is your pharmacist. A pharmacist is more than someone who is there to just sell you drugs. Pharmacists are highly trained and certified professionals who can take a look at what you have been prescribed and help you take the new prescription in a proper way and what to be aware of regarding side effects. Your pharmacist should also be able to evaluate any potential difficulties or concerns with drug combinations for your new prescription and what you have just been given by your physician and inform you in a clear and timely way regarding what to expect from drug combinations. At the very least, your pharmacist can help you avoid debilitating side effects from a drug combination, and, at the worst, help you avoid a situation that can seriously acerbate your condition and hurt your general health. Take the time to get to know your pharmacist similar to how you would get to know your physician and rely on him or her to help you avoid difficult situations.

There are two ways you can easily find out about drug combination effects. One is to use literature provided by your physician regarding the new prescription. This information should be given to you when you are initially given your prescription and encourage you to read it carefully and discuss any concerns with your physician or pharmacist. Another way that is growing in popularity is to look up the effects and drug combination concerns over a medication online. Most pharmaceutical companies have Websites with information regarding their drugs, you may also find general Websites on drugs and drug combinations that are not tied into a specific company.

Pain killers that are designed to help with a condition or work in combination with other drugs, sometimes available over-the-counter rather than by prescription, can be easily abused and cause significant health effects. Internal bleeding, hypertension and dependence can be easily caused by the misuse of pain killers, especially those using codeine. The same can be said for muscle relaxants such as valium or to sleep medications, which again, can be acquired without a prescription. Similar to prescriptions for specific conditions, pain killers should be thoroughly understood and used with the proper instructions.

Based on your own limited knowledge of your condition and your own feelings about your illness, you may be tempted to combine drugs in ways that were not intended when they were created or prescribed for you. This type of self-experimentation should be avoided at all costs. This does not mean you should not discuss your own ideas with your physician, but you need to recognize that any time you decide to medicate yourself in ways that were not initially prescribed, you should carefully review your ideas and plans with your physician before proceeding with actions that could cause you great harm. Communication for any reason regarding your treatment and prescription is key to safely and effectively using your prescription to treat your medical condition.

The Resources

Visit the following Websites for more information on drug treatment combinations:

Annals of Internal Medicine, *www.annals.org*

I Base, *www.i-base.info/guides*

BBC, *www.bbc.co.uk/1/hi/health*

Drug Library, *www.druglibrary.org*

BMJ Journals, *www.bmj.bmjournals.com*

Dot Now, *www.dotnow.org*

Drug Digest, *www.drugdigest.org*

Several books can be very helpful in learning about drug treatment conditions such as:

Combination Treatment of AIDS (Birkhauser Basel, 2003)

Drug Treatment in Old Age Psychiatry (Informa Healthcare, 2002)

Drug Treatment: What Works? (Routledge, 2004)

Best Pills, Worst Pills: A Consumer's Guide to Avoiding Drug-Induced Death or Illness (Pocket, 2005)

Drug Resistance in Oncology (CRC, 1997)

Drugs of Abuse and Immune Function (CRC Press, 1990)

Changes in Addiction Treatments

The Challenge

Not many years ago treating addictions, whether to alcohol or drugs, involved prolonged stays in a regular hospital facility, or even an asylum that specialized in the treatment of addictions. In some cases, addicts were tied to beds, allowed to detox and then observed and sent back into society. The root causes of the addictions were ignored for the sake of treating the obvious symptoms. The results of this type of treatment are not hard to imagine: addicts usually relapsed and either reentered the hospital or faced the very real possibility of dying from their addictions. In the mid 20th century, organizations such as Alcoholics Anonymous began looking at addiction as a disease that could be treated through participation in support groups and 12 step programs that recognized the nature of the addiction and how a reliance on a higher power could help fight the addiction. This model is now prevalent in addiction treatments and addictions are seen in a different light where the addict is not viewed as weak but as sick. This change has offered new hope to addicts. The challenge is to communicate these approaches to addicts and their families and making sure addicts are supported in their effort to save their lives.

The Facts

Alcoholics Anonymous (AA) is viewed frequently as the pioneer in a new type of addiction treatment, although the concepts behind the program have been around since the late 1930's. AA's approach is to let addicts know they are not alone, that everyone involved in the program has gone through similar experiences and that the treatment involves self-introspection and other important elements that have nothing to do with entering a hospital.

- Attending regular meetings of groups of similar addicts who openly discuss their experiences in a non-judgmental atmosphere;
- using a 12-step program to systematically address and deal with the addiction;
- acquiring a sponsor who can help the addict through the program and step in to work with an addict who is in danger of relapsing and
- an emphasis on spirituality or a higher power to turn to for help in dealing with an addiction.

Numbers of addicts in the United States are hard to accurately calculate. But, in 2004 it was estimated by the National Institute on Drug Abuse (NIDA) that 22.5 million Americans age 12 and over were in need of treatment for substance abuse. Of these, less than four million actually received treatment.

Untreated addictions carry a heavy cost beyond the emotional and personal financial impact to addicts and their families. Costs of addictions include those related to violent crime and property crime, expenses for imprisonment, healthcare costs, foster care and welfare costs and reduced work productivity. The most current estimate by the NIDA of these costs add up to a staggering $181 billion per year. The value in effective treatment on a financial basis is startling. For every dollar spent on effective addiction treatment programs, it is estimated there is are four dollar to seven dollar reductions in the cost of drug related crimes. In the case of some programs, total savings can reduce costs by a ratio of 12:1.

Drug addiction recovery is a long-term solution and not a short-term fix. Recovery can usually mean repeated episodes of treatment. Research into addiction treatments reveal several key elements have been shown to be vital in the treatment of drug or alcohol addiction.

- Individuals require individual approaches in treatment.
- Treatment needs to be readily available.
- Treatment needs to look at the complete needs of the individual and not just the addiction.
- Treatments need to be flexible, examined and reshaped to meet the needs of the addict.
- An addict has to commit to the treatment and stay in a program for the long term.
- Any effective treatment requires counseling and not just addressing physical health issues, although medications may be used to help alleviate the effects of the addiction.
- Addicts may have other mental conditions that need to be individually addressed.
- Medical treatment of withdrawal is only one aspect of treatment and will fade over time.
- Addiction treatment does not have to be voluntary. Interventions by family or friends of the addict may be necessary.
- Other diseases need to be detected as part of a drug addiction including HIV/AIDS, hepatitis B and C, tuberculosis and other infectious diseases.
- Recovery is a long-term process and may require ongoing or multiple episodes of treatment. Attending groups like AA could be a commitment for the rest of the addict's life.

Although most treatment programs involve treating the psychological aspects of the addiction, there are new drugs that can help with alleviating the withdrawal from the drug or alcohol and moving on with treatment of the addiction. Treating withdrawal is not an end in itself, but actually a starting point in treating the addiction.

- Methadone can be used to affect the same targets in the brain that opiates, such as heroin, affect.
- Buprenorphine is a relatively new treatment medication. These drugs are sometimes called Subutex or, in combination with naloxone, Suboxone. Under the Drug Addiction Treatment Act (DAT) of 2000, the United States Congress passed legislation that permit qualified physicians to prescribe narcotic medications to treat addictions. This allows addicts to acquire medication in a medical setting rather than a specialized clinic.

The Solutions

Addiction treatment's ultimate goal is to allow the individual addict to achieve lasting goals of sobriety. But, there are immediate goals in the treatment of the addiction that need to be addressed. These include a reduction or elimination of drug abuse, improvement in the functionality of the addict and minimization of the medical and social complications of drug or alcohol abuse. People in treatment for drug addiction are now taught to change their behavior to adopt a more healthy lifestyle.

Effective treatment involves both medication and behavioral therapy starting with detoxification and moving on to treatment and relapse prevention. Easing withdrawal symptoms can be crucial in the initial treatment and preventing relapse is vital. A relapsed addict may have to start over in a treatment program. New addiction treatments involve a continuum of care that address all aspects of a patient's life.

Outpatient behavioral treatment for drug addiction involves a wide variety of programs available to addicts at special clinics. Most of these programs involve individual or group counseling. Other programs offer different types of behavioral treatments.

- Cognitive Behavioral Therapy helps patients identify, avoid and cope with the situations where they are most likely to use drugs or alcohol.
- Multidimensional Family Therapy addresses teen drug addictions and is worked by the teen and his or her family.
- Motivational Interviewing seeks to identify the readiness of addicts to change their behavior and start treatment.
- Motivational Incentives uses positive reinforcement to encourage drug or alcohol abstinence.

Residential programs can be helpful for people with severe addictions. Therapeutic communities (TCs) have patients remain at a residence for six to 12 months. Some TCs are being adapted to deal with women who are pregnant or have children to care for.

The criminal justice system is looking more and more to address addictions. This is particularly true when the treatment program involves having the patient return to normal society. The treatment does not have to be voluntary to be effective. Studies from the Substance Abuse and Mental Health Services Administration indicate these types of treatments can cut drug abuse by half, reduce future criminal activity by 80 percent and reduce arrests for addiction-related crimes by up to 64 percent.

The Resources

Visit the following Websites for more information on addiction treatment:

Alcoholics Anonymous, *www.alcoholics-anonymous.org*

National Institute on Drug Abuse, *www.nida.nih.gov*

Medical News Today, *www.medicalnewstoday.com*

GreenFacts, *www.greenfacts.org*

National Institute on Alcohol Abuse and Alcoholism, *www.,niaaa.nih.gov*

Addiction Treatment Forum, *www.atforum.com*

Several books can be very helpful in explaining addiction treatments such as:

Addiction Treatment: A Strengths Perspective (Wadsworth Publishing, 2003)

The Addiction Treatment Planner (Wiley, 2005)

Substance Abuse Treatment and the Stages of Change: Selecting and Planning Interventions (The Guilford Press, 2004)

Seven Tools to Beat Addiction (Three Rivers Press, 2004)

Addictions: Concepts and Strategies for Treatment (Aspen Publishers, 1994)

Proven Holistic Treatment for Addiction & Chronic Relapse (Tate Publishing, 2006)

Section Three:

The Human Factor

26

Dealing with Nurse Practitioners

The Challenge

You may not need a doctor for all medical purposes. More and more busy physicians are using nurse practitioners (NPs) to handle some basic duties that do not involve complicated diagnoses or prescriptions for medication or therapies. The physician will still evaluate the patient and come up with a treatment program, the nurse practitioner will take care of monitoring, answering basic questions and referring the patient to the doctor when needed. A nurse practitioner may visit house-bound patients or see them in the doctor's office. They can act as a vital conduit between patient and physician and save each time and effort. This frees up the doctor for other important duties and allows the patient flexibility in scheduling appointments to monitor ongoing conditions. The challenge is to recognize what a nurse practitioner can and cannot do and taking utmost advantage of the service.

The Facts

There a variety of duties a NP can perform.

- Diagnosing, treating, evaluating and managing acute and chronic illness;
- taking medical histories and performing basic examinations;
- performing diagnostic studies and evaluating the results;
- prescribing some medications;
- helping with rehabilitation programs such as physical therapy;
- helping with prenatal and family planning services;
- performing annual physicals;
- doing minor surgeries and procedures such as skin biopsies, casting and suturing;
- providing referrals to physicians and
- counseling patients on healthy living and care.

There are many positive aspects to using nurse practitioners. According to the Academy of Nurse Practitioners:

- NPs bring expertise in counseling, patient education and case management skills to meet the growing demands of preventive medical care.

- NPs on average earn 40 percent less than a physician (depending on experience and area of specialization), thus saving the patient and the physician on treatment.
- Clinical outcomes for patients treated by NPs appear to be positive. A recent study by Journal of the American Medical Association found no significant difference in the health care status of ambulatory patients who were cared for by a NP or physician.

Most states require the initial diagnosis and plan of treatment be created by the physician. The NP then helps carry out this plan. You can examine the employment agreement between the NP and physician to see if there are any potential problems.

Aging patients may benefit most from the care of a NP. The NP can provide the proper combination holistic, thorough and preventive approach that older patients can benefit from. The NP often has a better bedside manner than a physician and is more willing to spend the time necessary to answer a patient's questions and concerns.

Nurses are still perceived as servants to physicians, but NPs are much more and often go through at least four years of training to acquire their NP credentials.

Most Registered Nurse (RN) training is similar to NP training and can lead to an RN moving on to be a NP. Like physicians, some NPs specialize in certain areas.

- Family NPs;
- pediatric NPs;
- adult NPs;
- geriatric NPs;
- women's health care NPs;
- neonatal NPs;
- acute care NPs;
- occupational health NPs;
- certified nurse midwives and
- certified nurse anesthetists.

RNs and NPs are among the fastest growing job categories in the country. This gives you more choices in using a NP, but also means you may not get the fit you need right away. Most NPs and RNs have to acquire a master's or associates degree or graduate from a certification program. Not all of these are created equally and you need to evaluate where the NP received his or her training.

The Solutions

Patients under NP care must recognize that billing to Medicare can be more challenging. Physicians have to follow separate guidelines for billing Medicare for NPs and this adds another layer of difficulty to the billing process.

Some NPs own their own practices, others work for a physician. You need to understand the scope of the collaboration between NP and physician.

The basic part of communication between NP and physician is the incident to the physician's services. This documents what was done by the NP and how it relates to the plan of treatment. It can give you an idea of what is being told your physician.

Using a nurse practitioner means freeing the physician from some visits, but the physician must still see the patient on a regular basis. At the same time, a physician must be present in the same office suite as the NP even if he or she does not actually see the patient.

Many patients believe only the physician can provide an accurate diagnosis, but NPs frequently are just as good at making the necessary observations and judgment. According to the *Journal of the American Medical Association*, NPs achieve comparable patient outcomes to that of a physician.

A good relationship with your NP is just as important as your relationship with your physician. Perhaps more so in that you will likely see a NP more often and spend more time with him or her. The relationship is based on communication, trust and understanding what a NP can or cannot do. The NP must know how you are feeling. You must believe you are receiving reliable advice and not have any false expectations on what the NP is allowed. You do this by asking questions and taking the time do the necessary follow-up. If possible, ask for references to find out a patient dealt with the NP.

Besides evaluating a patient condition and communicating that with the physician a NP, a NP can plan post-treatment home-care needs, diet and exercise programs, self administration of medications and physical therapy. Some NPs can help with grief therapy issues.

A NP must prove he or she has graduated from a bachelor or master's program in nursing or a special program that follows the formal education. The NP must also show the appropriate licensing. The license period may vary by state with some requiring biennial or triennial licensing. You should ask to see this proof before you decide to work with a NP.

While you may believe you are receiving a more accurate diagnosis and treatment program from a physician, you should recognize a NP can offer many of these services and spend more time with you than a physician.

You can work with NPs in a variety of settings, available in almost all states.

- Nurse managed health centers and community health care centers;
- public health departments;
- health maintenance organizations (HMOs);
- hospitals and clinics;

- hospice care centers;
- offices specifically for NPs;
- nursing homes and
- nursing schools including universities.

There are two basic parts of choosing a NP.

- Tangible proof of training and licensing and
- intangibles such as your perception you can comfortably work with this person.

You can change your mechanic or hair stylist. You can also change your NP if you believe the fit is not working, Your NP may be unaware of the problem, so you should take the time to explain your concern, give the NP a chance to respond and do not be too hasty in making a change. Remember, you will be starting from scratch with a new NP.

The Resources

Visit the following Websites for more information on nurse practitioners:

American Academy of Nurse Practitioners, *www.aanp.org*

American Nurses Association, *www.nursingworld.org*

All Business, *www.allbusiness.com*

The National Organizations of Nurse Practitioners, *www.nonpf.com*

Medscape, *www.medscape.com*

Center for Nursing Advocacy, *www.nursingadvocacy.org*

Nurse Practitioner Central, *www.npcentral.net*

Several books can be very helpful in helping you work with a nurse practitioner such as:

Practice Guidelines for Family Nurse Practitioners (W.B. Saunders, 1997)

Clinical Decision Making for Nurse Practitioners: A Case Study Approach (Lippincott, Williams and Wilkins, 1998)

Procedures for Nurse Practitioners (Lippincott, Williams and Wilkins, 2000)

Core Skills for Nurse Practitioners: A Handbook for Nurse Practitioners (Wiley, 2002)

27

Finding Medical Information

The Challenge

Sometimes a little knowledge can be dangerous thing, and when you acquire information about your medical condition, you may be causing yourself more worry than necessary. But, forewarned can also be forearmed and by learning about your condition you can better interact with your doctor and help you make informed choices about the nature of your condition and how you will approach the treatment. This information can help you understand your condition and, hopefully, feel more comfortable in how you are dealing with it. The information may be clinical in nature and discuss your specific condition, it may deal with broad issues in medical treatment or it may direct how you work with your physician and what relationship to strive for. The challenge is to find the information you need in a format you can easily use, evaluate it for its relative value and then know what to do with the information you receive. You can use the wealth of medical information available in a positive way as long as you understand its value and how best to use it.

The Facts

Many times the most obvious place to find current and relevant medical information is to search through the various organizations that specialize in disseminating medical information to the general public. In many cases, this information will be through professional support organizations for various specialties or types of diseases. There are many of these to choose from, but the easiest way to find links to most of these organizations is through the American Medical Association, *www.ama-assn.org* or through the United States government's Department of Health and Human Services, *www.hhs.gov*.

Worthwhile medical information online will often contain links or recommendations for further reading on your condition. This information may be on a related Website, article or book. By doing a little extra research on the recommendation, you can decide if it is worth your time to pursue this additional information.

One of your most effective tools in finding medical information online is through a reliable search engine. The most reliable are Google and Yahoo. These sites are relatively easy to use and can provide links to literally millions of possible Websites. To use them you simply type in the key words you are using to find information and evaluate the Website links that appear. Some of these links will contain free information, others will have information you may have to pay for, or are selling books or videos. The good search engines will show the most pertinent search results early on in the list, but it is worth your time to look past the first page of a Web search to make sure you are not missing any important information.

Besides medical information Websites, there are databases you can research medical information. Most of these you will have to access through your library. They include MEDLINE/PubMed or the Cumulative Index to Nursing and Allied Health Literature. Infotrac is a CD-ROM computer database that may prove useful. Many of the databases will have abstracts that summarize each journal article.

Besides public libraries, you can also use medical libraries to find information. Some of these libraries are linked to specific learning centers such as universities or medical schools. The books available often cannot be checked out, but the libraries should have coin-operated copiers available to copy the information you need. Some of the information may be on microfilm or microfiche. The librarian can help you use this equipment, which can also make hard copies.

Your friends may be able to point out worthwhile sources of good medical information that they have successfully used. A good physician can make the same type of recommendations. Be sure to use this information as a guide to further searching for information and judge the information on your own experience and your own needs. There are also groups online that share the latest in information regarding your condition. Reliable blogs, or Weblogs, may also be helpful to you, but remember to consume this information with an appropriate amount of skepticism and cross-check any information that does not seem quite right to you.

The Solutions

Taking your medical information to your appointments and asking questions may lead you to take the step toward finding a second opinion. You may not be getting the information you want to go with what you already know, or the answers you get may not agree with what you have been learning. At this point, it may be worth your time and effort to seek out and evaluate a second opinion.

There are several main methods to finding information regarding your medical condition or those of a friend or family member:

- Through your local public or professional library, often with the help of a good professional librarian;
- professional journals for various medical organizations available by contacting the medical organization or finding it in the periodicals department of your local library;

- books on your condition either available through your library or for purchase at your local bookstore or via Websites such as Amazon.com, www.amazon.com and
- Websites for various types of conditions from medical centers, university medical schools or from professional organizations.

Approach finding and learning medical information the same way you would digest information for a school project. This means using a highlighter or pen to make notes in the text of what you are reading, printing out the most important information from the Websites or taking notes on a separate pad of paper. Using notes will help you take the information you are learning to your next physician appointment to help you ask important questions.

Medical directories, available through your library or from a bookseller, can be effective ways to find medical information from other sources. The most popular of these directories include:

- Directory of Physicians in the United States, published by the American Medical Association and including vital information on physicians who are members of AMA;
- Health Hotlines, a booklet of toll-free numbers of health information hotlines from the National Library of Medicine or at www.sis.nlm.nih.og/hotlines;
- The official ABMS Directory of Board Certified Physicians which carries information on physicians certified in various specialties by the American Board of Medical Specialists;
- The Consumer Health Information Sourcebook and
- The Self-Help Sourcebook: The Comprehensive Reference of Self-Help Group Resources

Not only can you find information regarding medical conditions, you can also find the latest information on toxic or infectious problems through several easily used databases.

- Hazardous Substances Databank, HSDB, is a comprehensive, scientifically-reviewed, factual database containing records for over 4,500 toxic or potentially toxic chemicals:
- Toxlline contains references to literature on biochemical, pharmacological, physiological and toxicological side effects of drugs and other chemicals;
- HAZ_MAP which has references to occupational exposure to hazardous materials;
- Tox Town containing references to toxic chemicals and environmental health risks you may encounter in everyday life and everyday places and
- Household Products Databasee which addresses potential health effects, safety and handling of products in the home or garage.

There are several caveats to keep in mind as you find information regarding your medical condition. Knowing these common sense warnings may help you avoid misunderstanding the information you are receiving.

- Do not believe everything you read. Just because information is published online or in hard copy does not necessarily mean it is accurate or relevant.

- Compare different resources on the same topic to make sure you are not receiving conflicting information.
- Use your gut instinct whether the information rings true to you or not.
- Check the references at the end of the book or Web citation.
- What is the sources of your information. Look for a list of editorial or review board members or whether the information is peer-reviewed.
- Information reported in the mass media such as newspapers, popular magazines or large unreviewed Websites may be the least reliable.

The Resources

Visit the following Websites for more information on finding reliable medical information and how to use it:

American Medical Association, *www.ama.assn.org*

United States Department of Health and Human Services, *www.nih.org*

About Searching the Web for Medical Information, *www.about.com*

Health Insurance, *www.healthinsurance.about.com*

National Institute of Arthritis and Musculoskeletal and Skin Diseases, *www.niams.hig.gov*

Pavillion, *www.pavillion.co.uk*

Talking with Your Doctor, *www.nlm.nih.gov/medlineplus/talkingwithyourdoctor*

Several books can be very helpful in finding and using medical information such as:

The Merck Manual of Medical Information, Second Edition (Merck, 2003)

Understanding Medical Information: A User's Guide to Informatics and Decision-Making (McGraw-Hill Medical, 2001)

How to Find Medical Information on the Internet: A Print and Online Tutorial for the Healthcare Professional and Consumer (Library Associations Press, 1998)

American Medical Association Complete Guide to Your Children's Health (Random House, 1998)

A Senior's Health Journal: a Personal Record of Vital Health and Medical Information (St. Martin's Griffin, 2002)

After Any Diagnosis: How to Take Action Against Your Illness Using the Best and Most Current Medical Information Available (Three Rivers Press, 2001)

28

Finding the Right Fit for a Physician

The Challenge

Until we reach a certain age or develop a worrisome medical condition, most of us do not have a regular physician. Now it may be time to find a good physician who you can work with and feel confident in. This is a very important decision, but unfortunately many of us will spend more time choosing a car rather than making the effort to find a physician. You probably will not look for a discount doctor, but you may not be willing to spend the time to get the right fit from one of the most important professionals in your life. Luckily, there are a variety of criteria to examine and search methods to use before deciding on a physician. At the point where it comes down to making the final choice, you may end up relying on a so-called gut feeling that this the right fit. You can always change physicians, but this can be a major chore. So, making the initial right choice becomes that much more important.

The Facts

Not all doctors are created equally. Some are more competent than others. Some have a better bedside manner and communication by taking enough time to answer your questions. You need to evaluate these factors when you make your initial visit and do not be afraid to keep looking around if you are uncomfortable with the fit.

In most cases when you choose a physician that person will be a Primary Care Physician (PCP). They used to be called general practitioners. The PCP will evaluate your current medical condition and refer you to specialists as needed. Some PCPs also specialize in an area of medicine. Often, under current insurance plans, you will not be reimbursed for specialist treatment without a written referral from your PCP.

There are several methods of choosing a physician that go beyond find-a-doctor services or simply consulting the Yellow Pages.

- Ask friends and relatives for recommendations on what physicians they use and what their experiences have been.
- If you are moving to a new location ask your PCP for a recommendation for a physician in the area you are planning to relocate to.

- Use the referral services of your local hospitals.
- Check with your county's medical society. They can give you the name of several physicians who are accepting new patients.

You can find the qualifications of your physician by checking the Directory of Physicians in the United States, the Directory of Board Certified Physicians in your state's medical directory. The qualifications will include where the physician attended medical school, where he or she did their residence training, board certification, hospital affiliations and type of practices. This information can be found at your local library. You can also call the American Board of Medical Specialties at 800.776.2378 to verify the information.

You should have a comfortable enough relationship with your PCP to be able to discuss almost anything with him or her. This can include physical as well as emotional issues including possible alcohol or drug addiction. Trusting your PCP will help your basic care-routine well exams, preventive care and treatments for some illnesses or injuries go that much easier and smoothly.

Keep language requirements in mind as you choose a physician. You may need to be careful in finding a physician who can also speak languages such as Spanish or Polish. If you are bilingual helping out someone who only speaks a non-English language, you may need to be present during consultations to help with translating.

Do you believe your physician is spending adequate time with you after an examination? A good physician should be willing to spend time answering questions and not hurrying to the next examination. You can help keep a physician in the exam room for consultation, but, if you believe this is requiring an extraordinary effort, it may be time to make a change. Remember, the physician works for you, not the other way around.

The academic history of your physician does not mean he or she has to be a graduate of a high-profile under-graduate or medical school. Any certified medical school will follow similar educational procedures and have similar education requirements. A doctor with a sub-specialty should have received three to seven years of additional training in that specialty.

The Solutions

Take the time to write down what you are looking for in a physician before you start contacting potential PCPs. This will help you define your ideal doctor type and make your choice easier.

After you acquire, from whatever source or sources seem appropriate, the names of potential physicians, there is some checking you can do either before your first appointment or after you have made your initial visit.

- Do not assume the physician is properly licensed. Contact your state's office of professional registration or education department to find out about whether your physician is licensed. The education department should also be able to tell you where your physician received his or her education.
- Look beyond the physician to how the office is operated and its appearance.. What are the hours and locations, payment requirements, emergency and after-hours coverage and how the physician handles telephone consultations or home visits. Find out what hospitals the physician has admitting privileges. Evaluate how office staff answer your questions and communicate with the physician. Paperwork should be easy to fill out and self-explanatory.
- What is the physician record of being disciplined? You can call 800.663.6114 to find this out or visit your state's professional or educational Web sites. You will only find final disciplinary actions. Pending or dismissed actions are not part of the public record.

A major factor in choosing a physician may be the office's physical location and how convenient it is to your home or place of business. Most physicians schedule appointments Monday through Friday during the day. Saturday appointments may also be available but could be harder to schedule.

Are you more comfortable with a female or male physician? Discussing health care issues is a very personal process and many patients have their own feelings about gender. Do not assume men feel comfortable with men and women with women. It can depend on other psychological factors and areas of trust and comfort.

Carefully review whether your health insurance will cover a physician before moving forward in acquiring one. Insurance companies will publish names of physicians who qualify for the plan, or make their names available online. Double check with the physician's office when you make your initial appointment to make sure the physician still participates in the plan.

Always be honest with your PCP. He or she is not there to judge you or your behavior, but help in establishing and maintaining your health. In most cases, there is little your PCP has probably not heard and should be able to deal with your concerns honestly.

Look for fellowships, a form of recognition a physician will receive from his or her peers. This fellowship usually recognizes research or other intellectual endeavors. A fellowship is often listed on the physician's business card such as MC, FACS, standing for Medical Doctor, Fellow of the American College of Surgeons.

Trust your feelings when you meet your doctor. If it does not seem right for you for specific or less defined reasons, the relationship is probably not going to work. A good PCP should not appear to be judgmental, but honest and supportive in helping you with health issues.

The Resources

Visit the following Websites for more information on finding the right physician..:

American Medical Association's Doctor Finder, *www.ama.org*

Providence Health Systems, *www.providence.org*

Sutter Health, *www.sutterhealth.org*

Lifetime TV, *www.lifetimetv.com*

Medicine Net, *www.,medicinenet.com*

Ask Men, *www.askmen.com*

Several books can be very helpful in helping select the right physician for you such as:

Communication in Medical Care: Interaction Between Primary Care Physicians and Patients (Cambridge University Press, 2006)

Choosing Assistive Devices: A Guide of Users and Professionals (Jessica Kingsley Publishers, 2002)

The Physician: The Cultivation, Education, Duties, Standards of Behavior and Judiciousness of the Physician (BookSurge Publishing, 2006)

Choosing Wisely: How Patients and Their Families Can Make Right Decisions About Life and Death (Image, 1992)

How to Choose Your Family Doctor and Keep Him (Exposition Press, 1974)

How to Choose A Good Doctor (Andover Publishing Group, 1979)

29

Using Recommendations and Find-A-Doctor Services

The Challenge

Depending on where you live there are probably a large number of physicians to choose from. This starts with the choice of a primary care physician whether a general practitioner or an internist. Because of ethics rules you will not find blatant advertising regarding a physician beyond location, phone number, specialty, education background and how many years the physician has been practicing. This information can be accessed through Websites regarding what physicians are available to you in your area. Often the physician's information will be available by calling the physician's office and asking some basic questions. You can then use this information to compare physicians and help you make an informed choice on who you might wan to visit. Sometimes this information is available through find-a-doctor services made available online or through a clearinghouse operated by your local medical society or state medical agency. You can also take a low-tech approach by simply talking to friends and family regarding who they are using as a physician, what the nature of the relationship is and how they feel about their physician. Sometimes this recommendation is based on aspects that do not involve empirical information but, rather, a feeling for the physician and matching that with what you need. Choosing a physician can be challenging and needs to involve some homework from you. The challenge is to recognize how you feel about physicians in general, what you are looking for both practically and in terms of a feel for your physician, using the right mechanisms to find a physician and combining all that information into a matrix that can help you make a good choice for you. While you can always change your physician after you have been working with him or her for some time, it is easier and more productive to find the right physician in the beginning and staying with that person. By using the tools available you can find a good physician for you.

The Facts

As it has for many areas of life, using online services to help you find a physician has revolutionized the process. You can visit a Website operated by your local medical society or state medical organization and use this Website to help you locate a physician who is a good practical fit. Most of these Websites are designed to be as easy to use as possible. You should be able to input standard search criteria into a search engine. If you leave this section as No Preference, you will probably receive a listing of all physicians in your area. You can search by name of the physician, based on other information you have already received, by searching manually for a name or searching by the first letter of the physician's last name. In most cases searching by name will return a list of all physicians with a certain alphabetical sequence at the beginning of the name. For example making an entry like Smi will probably return listings for Smith, Smithson, Smitty and other similar names.

One of the best examples of a Website that is not operated by a local medical society or state medical agency is the Website operated by the popular WebMD. This Website offers you the chance to locate a physician in your area with a minimum of difficulty and in an intuitive way that can help you access the Website and allow you to use it very quickly and easily. The site begins by asking you what zip code city/state you are searching for. If you know this, you can search by the physician's last name. If you do not have a specific physician in mind you can search broad medical categories including cardiology, primary care physician or family physician, neurology, pediatrics, dermatology, gastroenterology, obstetrics/gynecology, vision, internal medicine, orthopedics and psychiatry. You can also choose from more specific or less used specialties. The Website does not allow you to use the information to set up advertising. It does not warrant the status of its information and urges you to find current information by further contacting the physician's office.

Using a Find-A-Doctor service or online scheduling does not mean you can directly access a specialist. In most cases, your primary care physician will need to refer you to a specialist. This is so you are visiting a specialist that can treat your condition and that your PCP has a good experience in working with in the past.

The Solutions

Any marketing professional will tell you the most effective method of choosing a product or service is through word of mouth. This means your family and friends can help point you in the right direction regarding what to use. If this method is effective in choosing laundry soap, it can also be effective in choosing a physician. You must be honest with your friends and family regarding why you are looking for a physician and what would be a good fit for you.

Once you know whether your friends or family are using a physician that might be a good fit for you, there are several questions you need to ask regarding their relationship with the physician.

- What is the name of the physician?
- Where is the physician located and is parking nearby an issue?
- What are the physician's office hours? Does the physician offer evening or weekend appointments?

- How easy is it to get an appointment?
- Is it possible to get an appointment at the last minute?
- Do you know if the physician is accepting new patients?
- How is the office staff and other support staff to work with?
- Do you feel comfortable using the physician and why?
- What do you feel are the strengths and weaknesses of the physician?

Each online service will have slight variations in how you will use them, but for the most part they will use the same basic mechanisms to help you locate and access a physician. If a physician is listed as working within the Find-A-Doctor system you are using, you should be able to use an online form to make your initial appointment. This form will have information marked with an asterisk that must be filled out. Usually the form will not send you an online confirmation, but you will receive a telephone call within a day confirming an appointment or giving you appointment options. Using an online appointment form will not guarantee you will be able to visit a physician at a certain time, you will usually receive a list of availabilities to choose from. Most online forms will allow you to call a phone number if you are having difficulty using the online service or would rather use a more traditional method.

A Find-A-Doctor service is customizable, convenient, time efficient and will help you stay informed. Most Find-A-Doctor services, whether using a phone tree or Website, has information that is updated on a daily basis, although it is always a good idea to call the physician ahead of time to make sure the information is correct. In general a good Find-A-Doctor service will help you find the following information:

- Physician name;
- physician phone number;
- specialty;
- age;
- gender;
- languages spoken in the office;
- office location and a map/directions to the office;
- physician education;
- physician certifications;
- practice profile indicating the way your case will be handled;
- professional affiliations and
- the types of insurance accepted.

Often your medical insurance carrier can help you find a physician who is working within their plan. This will help you make a choice that will expedite being reimbursed by your physician. Medicare can also help in Find-A-Doctor services, but may not be as up-to-date as your private medical insurance. This information is not a recommendation for the physician, but a listing of who is covered by your insurance.

The Resources

Visit the following Websites for more information on using recommendations and find-a-doctor services:

Alegent Services, *www.alegent.com*

Medicare, *www.medicare.gov*

American Association of Retired Persons, *www.aarp.org*

WebMD, *www.webmd.com*

Sharp, *www.sharp.com*

AMA Doctor Finder, *www.ama-assn.org/doctorfinder*

Doctor Directory, *www.doctordirectory.com*

Several books can be very helpful in learning about using recommendations and find-a-doctor services such as:

Your Body, Your Health: How to Ask Questions, Find Answers and Work with Your Doctor (Prometheus Books, 2002)

Healing Without Fear: How to Overcome Your Fear of Doctors, Hospitals, and the Health Care System and Find Your Way to True Healing (Healing Arts Press, 2002)

How Doctors Think: Clinical Judgment and the Practice of Medicine (Oxford University Press, 2005)

Doctors: The Biography of Medicine (Vintage, 1995)

Marketing for Therapists: A Handbook for Success in Managed Care (Jossey Bass, 1996)

American Medical Association Guide to Talking to Your Doctor (Wiley, 2001)

30

Not All Doctors Are Created Equally— When to Recognize A Bad Fit and How to Make A Change

The Challenge

Like all professional relationships you may work for some time with a physician and slowly realize the relationship is not working, This may depend on a variety of factors, both practical and a sense that this is simply not a good fit for you. You must understand that not all physicians are as competent as others or have the same type of people skills that will work with you. You know when you feel comfortable and this comfort may be based on no more than a feeling that the relationship is not working, Once you recognize that you have a bad fit with your physician, you must then recognize and understand what is the best way to make a change. This change can have profound effects on the quality of your medical care and should not be taken lightly. It is similar to finding a physician in the first place. The challenge is to recognize the reality of who your physician is and how he or she is working with you, how other aspects of the physician's practice works with you, when you must realize you are working in a non-productive environment and how to make a change in your present condition that is least disruptive to your medical care. With this realization and information you can maintain a vital approach to your medical care that stresses how the physician is working with you and not what you need to do to make the relationship work. You will find yourself free to make the changes you need and add to the alternatives available to you in your medical care.

The Facts

There are several reasons to look at changing your physician that may not be caused by recognizing if your current physician is not working out for you:

- You have just moved to a new area outside the convenient service area of your current physician.
- You have moved out what can be considered the service area of your current physician.
- Your current physician has moved into a new area.
- Your current physician, for any number of reasons, has removed you from the service list of patients.

Saying goodbye to your current physician can be difficult. Your decision may depend on insignificant details such as difficulty in parking, dealing with snippy office staff, having difficulty making an appointment and disliking the office décor. However, typically the reason you may want to make a change is because of the lack of chemistry with your current physician. Changing physicians due to a bad feeling about working with the physician can be an anxiety ridden process and there is no guarantee a new physician is going to work any better meeting your practical and emotional needs.

Many physicians will underestimate the importance of good patient communication and are often surprised when they lose a patient because they are simply not good communicators. Despite of what a physician may think of the importance of technical ability they do not understand the importance of rapport and communication. An American College of Physicians survey found that both patients and physicians rate technical ability as the most important factor to maintaining a relationship, but patients will rank communication as a number two reason to maintain a relationship, while physicians rank it number six.

The time when physicians do not care about the administrative side of the practice are long past. Anything that happens to you in the physician's office should be of concern to the physician. You need to let the physician know when the administrative side of the practice is not working for you and what you hope you can do to help correct the problem with the physician.

Pay attention to the practice group and its policies the same you would evaluating the individual performance of your physician. Practice groups tend to have their own sense of integrity and will bring in physicians who match their philosophy in treating patients. A recommendation regarding a physician should give you some idea of how the practice group does business.

Evaluating whether to change your physician and who to choose may depend on whether your physician is diversified enough to treat a variety of comorbid conditions, does your physician work with a good variety of colleagues and can you be assured there will be continuity of care if other physicians are called upon with the practice group.

The Solutions

You have the right to change your physician without giving the office a reason. The process of finding a new physician is similar to registering with your current physician. You do not have to, but it would be helpful to notify your current physician you are making a change. This will facilitate transferring your records to a new physician.

All patients are justifiably concerned with the technical ability and expertise of a physician. They assume their physician will be competent. How the physician interacts with the patient can shake that conviction. A patient needs to judge clinical knowledge and technical skills through the lens of the physician's interpersonal qualities.

Before you spend the time and effort to change physicians, spend time figuring out what bothers about your current relationship. You need to do some honest soul searching before determining if you have a bad fit and need to change physicians. The reasons for making the change usually include several factors:

- Is the physician's approach considered too dictatorial and does not allow the patient to have necessary input?
- Does the physician seem distracted or interrupts the appointment?
- Does your physician talk down to you?
- Does your physician confuse you with jargon?
- Can it take two days to get a phone call returned?
- Does it take weeks to get results from tests?

Attempting to work out difficulties with your physician is usually more worthwhile and a better use of your time than making a change. Share with your physician what is troubling you and how the physician can work better with you. Bring it up if you feel you are not receiving sufficient information from your physician. Let him or her know you are spending too much time sitting in the waiting room for you appointment. Bring any problems you are having with nurses or office staff to the attention of your physician. Describe any bad experiences with your physician during an appointment or write a letter of concern to your physician and mark the communication as personal.

Before making a change in your physician you should ask yourself whether your own expectations are reasonable. If you want your physicians to take and return phone calls immediately, you should expect the physician to interrupt your visit and take these calls from others.

Once you decide to change physicians, you should undergo a search process similar to finding your current physician. You may want to do online research or act on the recommendations of friends and family. If you are asking around, you need to find people with similar conditions to give you a recommendation.

The business end of the practice can be as important as dealing with the physician. These business practices fall under several areas:

- Does your physician make it easier for you to pay be accepting your co-pays or payments for other services with a credit card?
- Does your physician offer free samples of medication when this is appropriate?
- Is your physician part of the HMO you are currently participating in?
- Does your physician accept Medicare or Medicaid payments?
- Is your physician on a PPO list offered by your place of employment?

The Resources

Visit the following Websites for more information on recognizing a bad fit and changing physicians:

National Health Services in England, *www.nhs.uk/england/doctors/changedoctor*

American College of Physicians, *www.acponline.org*

About Arthritis, *www.arthritis.about.com*

Answers at Yahoo, *www.answers.yahoo.com*

You Are Able, *www.yourable.com*

Center for the Advancement of Health, *www.cfah.org*

Several books can be very helpful in learning to recognize a bad fit and changing physicians such as:

Health Care Providers, Institutions and Patients: Changing Patterns of Care Provision and Care Delivery (JAI Press, 2000)

A Marketing Approach to Physician Recruitment (Haworth Press, 1995)

The Changing Nature of Physician Power and Its Future (Journal of Power and Ethics, 2000)

The Continuing Professional Development of Physicians (American Medical Association Press, 2003)

Leading Physicians through Change: How to Achieve and Sustain Results (American College of Physician Executives, 2000)

Beyond Managed Care: How Consumers and Technology Are Changing the Future of Health Care (Jossey-Bass, 2000)

Section Four:

Finding Support

31

Development of Support Groups

The Challenge

Physicians and health care professionals are recognizing more and more that a vital part of employee recovery is to use the variety of support groups available, in some cases, for very specific elements of medicine. These support groups are not only important in the healing process but also for those patients who are coping with long-term illnesses that may not be substantially curable. These support groups can also be important for the families of patients who are dealing with catastrophic illnesses. In some cases, the families may be part of a support group with a patient, in others the family is involved in their own groups. In some cases, the support group may be offered through a hospital or other formal health care facility, in others the support group might be offered by a private organization that may be free or charge a nominal fee to the participant. The challenge is to understand the benefits or downsides to using a support group, what groups are available and in what setting and what a patient or family can reasonably expect from the support group. When used wisely, a good support group can be very beneficial in a patient's recovery and the family's ability to deal with a medical condition.

The Facts

Support groups are more than likely not run by a physician or even a licensed therapist. Those individuals will work with the patient and the family on a one-on-one basis. The support group is often run by a nurse practitioner or other similar type of caregiver. In many cases, the support group is run by a volunteer with experience with the medical condition, or as a family member of a patient dealing with a certain condition. The person leading the group may be do so on a rotating basis where different group members lead separate types of the group.

A support group may meet in a variety of locations including a hospital, medical care facility, church, community center or even someone's home. The key is to establish an area of mental comfort besides any physical comfort. This may include making available refreshments, such as coffee, water and snacks for the participants. Although most support groups do not charge a formal fee to attend the group, they may request a nominal voluntary contribution that helps pay for the rental of a space and for any refreshments.

It is important for any support group to maintain some level of confidentiality. This does not mean a participant should not share what is being experienced in the group, but avoids specific identification of who the person is and what the nature of their behavior or problems are. A good support group with an acceptable level of confidentiality, especially a support group for addicts, will normally use only a first name to identify the participant and will encourage all participants to not discuss aspects of the meetings with people who are not part of the support group.

An alternative to physically attending a support group is to use online newsgroups. These are also called Internet Discussion Groups and function like electronic worldwide bulletin boards. Using a discussion group allows you to reply to a posting talking to the entire list or just to the individual making the posting. There are literally hundreds of newsgroups to choose from with the challenge being finding the pertinent ones for you. A good starting point is visiting the Website Deja News, *www.dejanews. com,* which provides a comprehensive search of online newsgroups. You can also do a simple word search to locate an appropriate newsgroup. Remember, not all the information you will find on a newsgroup is correct and you should always consult your health care professional before acting on what you are reading.

The Solutions

One of the more prevalent forms of support groups are those that deal with addictive areas of a person's life. Although health issues may be involved in some of these groups, more often they are designed along a social element that help patients recognize the reality of their condition, what effect this condition is having on their lives and how others are dealing with similar issues. This type of support group may not offer any concrete answers on how to cure someone of an addiction, many addictions are not really curable and only can be coped with, but help patients find ways to avoid the type of destructive behavior they have been indulging in. These addictions can take many forms including alcohol, drugs such as cocaine or heroin, gambling, eating and even sexual. Some addiction support groups such as Al-Anon are not designed for the actual addict but were created to help family and friends deal with an alcoholic or drug addicted individual, help him or her find treatment and deal with their own conflicting feelings of being involved with an addict.

It is not unusual for a patient or addict to resist attending a support group because he or she perceives the group as being an unwelcome reminder of his or her condition or addiction. The real nature of the support group as a way to heal physically and mentally may not be properly understood, but when used properly, a good support group can be very beneficial. The key is to find the right type of support group and then be willing to actively participate in the efforts of the group. This means contributing to any discussion and sharing your own experiences as to how you are dealing with the condition. It means honestly listening to and evaluating what is being heard during meetings of the support group and acting on ideas that seem to fit in well with what you are experiencing. It means establishing a two-way street where what is being said by the participant is just as important as what is being heard.

There are a variety of methods to finding good support groups. Good referrals are based on either personal knowledge of those leading the group or the experiences of their participants. Ways to get these referrals include:

- Information provided by your health care provider including written information on a support group;
- material that is available for free on support groups and can be found at a hospital, clinic or other health care facility;
- Websites on medical support groups. These include a variety of resources such as the Directory of Online Genetic Support Groups, Genetic and Rare Conditions Site, Health Hotlines, Open Directory Project—Support Groups and the Self-Help Sourcebook Online.

Other common support groups available for physical and mental health issues include:

- Black Women's Support Group;
- Communication Skills;
- Creating Opportunities for Personal Effectiveness, COPE;
- Getting off the Rollercoaster Group;
- Graduate Student Group;
- Making Peace with Food Group;
- New Life After Midlife;
- Returning from Medical Leave Group;
- Skills for Effective College Living;
- Substance Abuse Recovery Group;
- All About Procrastination;
- Relaxation Training and
- Lesbian, Bisexual, Gay, Transsexual and Questioning Group.

If you cannot find an existing support group in your area that meets your needs, you might consider starting your own group. Before you take concrete action to begin a support group consider the following factors:

- What do you want your group to accomplish?
- Should your group be affiliated or registered with a national organization?
- How large do you want the group to be?
- How will you promote your group and attract new members?
- How will your group be funded?
- Why type of weekly or monthly meeting schedule do you want your group to have?
- Where can you hold your group meetings?
- Will your group have a formal structure or will participants just be able to attend and participate as they see fit?

As you form your own group, you may want to consider using a periodic outside speaker to address the group. Selecting the speaker may depend on your own experiences or from the recommendations of others with the same type of condition. Professionals are busy, but are usually willing to help a good support group. Make sure you properly promote any session using a speaker. An alternative to a speaker is taking your group on a field trip to a facility that relates to the condition being addressed by the group.

The Resources

Visit the following Websites for more information on forming or using medical support groups:

Jenkins Law, *www.jenkinslaw.org*

Massachusetts Institute of Technology, *www.web.mit.edu*

Geocities, *www.geocities.com*

Yahoo, *www.health.yahoo.com/groups*

Oreilly, *www.oreilly.com/medical*

Microsoft Network, *www.health.msn.com*

Daily Strength, *www.dailystrength.org*

Several books can be very helpful in forming or using medical support groups such as:

Major Incident Medical Management and Support: The Practical Approach to the Hospital (BMJ Publishing Group, 2005)

The Self-Help Group Sourcebook: Your Guide o Community & Online Support Groups (American Self-Help Group Clearinghouse, 2002)

Starting and Sustaining Genetic Support Groups (The Johns Hopkins University Press, 1996)

Special Incident Medical Management and Support: The Practical Approach (BMJ Publishing Group, 2007)

AIDS Trauma and Support Group Therapy: Mutual Aid, Empowerment, Connection (Free Press, 1996)

Self-Help Support Groups for Older Woman: Rebuilding Elder Networks Through Personal Empowerment (Taylor and Francis, 1997)

32

Integrating Mental Therapy In Physical Care

The Challenge

The science and medicine of mental therapy is usually considered its own discipline. It can be practiced by trained counselors/social workers, psychologists with a PhD degree and proper licensing or a psychiatrist with an MD who can also prescribe drugs as well as provide counseling. Many times patients will seek out these professionals to deal with a variety of issues from relationship concerns to depression to more serious conditions such as schizophrenia or bipolar disease. They can offer tremendous help in dealing with a variety of problems. However, more and more health professionals are recognizing the importance of incorporating mental therapy in the overall treatment of medical conditions that may not be specific to mental health care. Physicians have discovered that patients who maintain a proper mental attitude and work with a professional to understand the nature of their condition and the necessities of treatment can benefit more from common treatment. The mental therapy may include discussing why this condition has occurred and what it may ultimately mean to the quality of life for the patient. It may include recognizing the importance of a good attitude towards the condition and placing it in context of the patient's life and future. It can be tremendously therapeutic. The challenge is to understand the nature of what mental therapy can do to benefit your treatment for a physical condition, who to find to supply the appropriate counseling for you and what you need to do to help maintain a good mental attitude. By incorporating proper mental therapy, you can better deal with your physical condition, increase its effectiveness and help speed along the healing process. Using mental therapy is not a sign of weakness, but, rather a sign of strength where you have the courage and self-awareness to take advantage of all the therapeutic tools available to you and your physicians.

The Facts

Not only can you receive mental therapy from a specialist such as a psychologist or psychiatrist, you can also receive help from a mental therapy nurse. Psychiatric nursing works within nursing models and utilizes nursing care plans. It seeks to care for the entire person. The emphasis on mental health nursing is the development of a therapeutic relationship with the patient and understanding the nature of the patient's mental health as it affects the healing process of physical care. Developing this relationship means the mental therapy nurse must seek to engage with the patient in a positive and collaborative manner that helps empower patients to draw n inner resources as well as any other treatments they may be receiving.

The development of a therapeutic relationship with a mental health professional can present challenges that are not found during other types of physical therapies. The difficulty is not just because of the nature of the patient's mental health issues, but also because the patients may be initially developing the relationship in a psychiatric hospital and could be needed to receive treatments against their will. The therapist must also have a level of self-awareness to help understand and properly utilize the experience as it relates to physical therapies.

Psychosocial interventions are frequently used to help patients cope with physical treatment of a medical condition. The interventions are now mostly delivered by nurses in mental health settings and include cognitive behavioral therapy, family therapy to help the family deal with the patient's treatment and milieu therapy or psychodynamic approaches. The idea is to work with a patient over a period of time and use psychological methods to allow the patient to employ techniques he or she can use to aid recovery and help manage any future mental health crisis.

Mental health patients usually receive treatment in a standard variety of settings:

- A hospital, where patients can be voluntarily or involuntarily committed is generally used during a crisis that means they represent a danger to themselves or others. Mostly these stays are open-ended, but patients can admit themselves to a hospital for a set period of time to accomplish a specific goal.
- The patient's home can sometimes be a therapeutic setting. The emphasis is working on mental health promotion in a comfortable environment. The treatments are normally administered and monitored by mental therapy nurses. An offshoot of this is using outpatient rehabilitation centers.
- Elderly people are often treated in an environment that can help deal with specific age issues such as dementia. Adolescents undergoing mental issues are often also treated in facilities separate from those for adults.

The Solutions

Whether the mental therapy is received from a doctor or from a nurse the therapeutic relationship with the patient can be looked at in three distinct phases:

- Orientation phase is having the patient get to know the therapist and vice versa and clarifies the purpose of the relationship.
- Working phase is the period when the majority of the therapy work is performed.
- Resolution phase is where the patient in care becomes more independent and is eventually able to eventually end the therapeutic relationship.

Treatment for psychiatric difficulties usually fall into three distinct categories:

- Psychiatric or psychotropic medications is a very commonly used method of mental health interventions. Psychiatrists will prescribe drugs and they and the mental therapy nurses will help administer the medications either orally or through intra-venous injections. Side effects from the medication and their effect on the patient's attitudes will be closely monitored using standard assessments. The patient should receive detailed information on the medication to be used to make an informed choice on whether to use the medication or an alternative.
- Electroconvulsive therapy, sometimes commonly referred to as electroshock therapy, is somewhat controversial but can assist with the preparation and recovery from mental health therapy. The therapy usually is administered in a clinical setting and involves the use of a mild anesthesia.
- Physical care is used to ensure patients have acceptable levels of self-care, nutrition, sleep and other beneficial treatments. They are vital to tend to any concomitant physical ailments.
- Psychoanalysis, developed by Sigmund Freud, is the oldest form of psychotherapy. The patient usually relaxes in a comfortable setting four or five times a week and attempts to say whatever comes to mind in a practice called free association.
- Cognitive therapy and behavior therapy can be very helpful in helping deal with mental distress that relates to physical treatments. Cognitive therapy acts on the principle that how the patient feels and behaves is based on how they interpret their experiences. Identifying core beliefs and assumptions can help patients begin to think different ways about their medical experience. Behavior therapy is based on the idea that faulty methods of dealing with crisis is due to faulty learning in the past. Behavior therapy helps people let go of maladaptive behaviors.
- Hypnosis and hypnotherapy are somewhat controversial but can help patients deal with the discomfort and pain of medical treatments. It induces a trance that helps the patient relax and post-hypnotic techniques of continuing the therapies.

Besides clinical psychiatric methods, some patients are exploring spiritual interventions. These address spiritual crises by focusing on developing a sense of meaning, purpose and person for the patient undergoing physical care. Spiritual interventions are designed to strengthen the patient's relationship with a God or a higher power. Using meditation or prayer, this may be a religious or non-religious experience. Spiritual interventions stress engagements with the physical care problems and help family and friends be with the patient during a time of crisis rather than trying to fix the problem.

Instead of using mental health professionals, some patients can use alternative forms of self-help therapy. These include improving diet and nutrition, undergoing counseling from a clergyman, animal assisted therapies, art therapy, dance and movement therapy and music and sound therapy. Each has its place and successes.

Biofeedback, guided imagery and massage therapy are also possibilities for mental health therapies that can assist you deal with medical treatments.

The Resources

Visit the following Websites for more information on mental health and physical treatment:

Merck, *www.merck.com*

National Mental Health Information Center, *www.mentalhealth.samhsa.gov*

Healthy Place, *www.healthyplace.com*

Web MD Mental Health Center, *www.webmd.com/mentalhealth*

National Institute of Mental Health, *www,nimh.nih.gov*

Mental Health Net, *www.mentalhelp.net*

New York Online Access to Health, *www.noah-health.org*

Several books can be very helpful in learning about mental health and physical treatment such as:

Complementary and Alternative Treatments in Mental Health Care (American Psychiatric Publishing, 2006)

Geriatric Mental Health Care: A Treatment Guide for Health Professionals (The Guilford Press, 2001)

Getting Help: The Complete & Authoritative Guide to Self-Assessment and Treatment of Mental Health Problems (New Harbinger Publications, 2006)

Handbook of Multicultural Mental Health: Assessment and Treatment of Diverse Populations (Academic Press, 2000)

Homeopathic Medicine for Mental Health (Healing Arts Press, 1984)

Natural Mental Health: How to Take Control of Your Own Emotional Well-Being (Hay House, 2000)

Section Five:

Insurance

33

The Pros and Cons of Different Health Insurance Plans

The Challenge

One of the most potentially devastating financial costs to you and your family could be from medical expenses. These expenses could come from injury, unexpected illness or a planned procedure. The expenses will cover a wide variety of areas: costs for physician care, hospital stay, therapy even items as small as a bandage. Every item involved in a medical procedure can cost you and you will be responsible for paying these expenses in a timely manner. To offset these costs, many people will carry some type of medical insurance. This insurance is designed to pay a portion, or, in some cases, all of those expenses. Without health insurance, many people will put off medical treatment until the condition has progressed to a dangerous state and may be more difficult to treat. The challenge is to identify and understand any insurance plans offered by employers, what is available in private insurance, the differences between insurance plans and what you need to do to make sure you are getting the most value from your insurance.

The Facts

One of the ongoing debates regarding health care coverage is private insurance vs. universal coverage. This compares paying for your own insurance against using government approved health care providers. Currently the United States does not offer universal, or single-payer, coverage, however some foreign countries such as Canada or the United Kingdom do. You will usually not pay for services provided under universal coverage, but you will have less say in which physician you visit and may have to wait longer to see a physician. Some people who live in a country offering universal coverage purchase supplementary insurance to give them more say in what type of care they will receive.

When you become part of an insurance plan, whether it is a group plan offered from your employee or an individual plan you purchase yourself, you will usually receive an insurance card to fit into your wallet and a detailed explanation of your plan. This explanation may seem daunting, but you should take the time to read and understand what provisions are offered through your plan. The insurance card will carry vital information regarding your health insurance:

- Your name;
- your Social Security Number;
- the name of your health provider including whatever special name the plan may cover;
- the employee identification for you in the plan;
- the identification number for your plan and
- contact information for your provider including phone and fax numbers and Website.

Be sure to take your insurance card with you for your initial visit to a Primary Care Physician or specialist. The office staff will note the information and, in most cases, make a copy of the front and back of the card for their records.

After you receive a medical procedure outside a well-patient visit, the bill for the treatments you receive will be submitted to your insurance carrier for their determination, based on the specifics of your plan, on what they will pay and what will be your responsibility. Once this determination is made, it will be submitted to the health care provider who will issue you a bill. The information, called an Explanation of Benefits (EOB), will also be sent to you for your records. You should review this EOB carefully to make sure it is in keeping with how you interpret your plan, and contact your health care provider if you believe the EOB is in error.

The two most prevalent types of managed health-care plans are Health Maintenance Organizations (HMOs) and Preferred Provider Organizations (PPOs). Besides the differences in corporate structures between the two, there are several important differences you should be aware of when evaluating which type of system to use.

- Members of HMOs must choose a Primary Care Physician from the physician members of the HMO. The Primary Care Physician must be consulted to visit a specialist, who must also be a member of the HMO. Under a PPO you do not choose a Primary Care Physician and can refer yourself to a specialist.
- You will typically not receive coverage under an HMO for care received from non-network physicians. Under a PPO, you are not required to stay within a network, but you will probably be charged substantially more if you go outside the network. This can be as much as 20 percent of patient costs.
- You will probably not have to meet a deductible before your benefits begin under a HMO and instead will pay a nominal co-payment. PPOs often require you to meet a deductible, especially for hospitalization and may have larger co-payments than HMOs.

Your choices in health insurance often come down to choosing an individual plan over a group health insurance plan. A group plan means you are part of a specific group, which often is your workplace. It is usually less expensive to go for a group plan, but a group plan may offer you less choices in your care. Another factor to evaluate is whether your insurance plan will cover your family, usually by paying an extra monthly benefit either out-of-pocket or deducted from your paycheck.

Beyond standard HMOs or PPOs for health care insurance, there are several special type of health insurance plans you can evaluate, some for very specific needs.

- High deductible insurance plans are less expensive but can cost you more for the actual care;
- catastrophic insurance plans are for patients concerned about serious conditions such as a heart attack or stroke and go above normal insurance coverage;
- fee-for-service insurance has you a pay monthly fee to the plan and then for each service used;
- Medicare and Medicaid are government offered insurance plans for the elderly and those with financial need to help pay for their medical expenses;
- disability insurance covers loss of income in the vent of a long-term illness or recovery from injury when you cannot work;
- hospital indemnity insurance pays a fixed amount for hospital stays up to a maximum amount of days; and
- long-term care insurance covers the cost of a nursing home or in-home care which can easily add up to thousands of dollars per month.

The Solutions

Many insurance plans encourage well-patient visits. These are regular visits and examinations by a Primary Care Physician and are usually available for a small payment by the member of the insurance plan, usually between ten and 30 dollars per visit. Sometimes these visits are totally paid for by the plan. The purpose of paying for most of these well-patient visits is to identify medical conditions before they turn into major expenses. After the age of 40, most people are encouraged to take advantage of these well-patient visits, and, of course they should be done if the member of the plan believes he or she has a medical condition that should be evaluated by a Primary Care Physician.

Be aware of what physicians and dentists are approved by your health insurance plan. In most cases, health insurance plans will not include every physician or dentist. If your care provider is not covered by your plan, you will not be reimbursed for any portion of the cost of care. Most health insurance providers will publish printed material listing what Primary Care Physicians or specialists are covered by your plan. This information may also be available online. You may want to call a potential physician prior to a visit to make sure he or she is covered by the plan.

Most insurance plans are structured to be driven by a Primary Care Physician. This means they will not cover a procedure by a specialist unless specifically referred to a specialist by the Primary Care Physician. This recommendation will become part of your patient record. You will usually be issued a written referral statement indicating what condition is supposed to be evaluated by the specialist. This referral should be given to your specialist when you arrive for the evaluation.

When deciding on an insurance plan, you should look at important factors and options before deciding on the plan.

- How many physicians are covered and how convenient are they located for your use?
- What is your out of pocket deductible costs, costs that you will have to pay for physician visits or health care?
- What percentage of your costs will be paid by the plan after you meet your deductible costs?
- What services are provided by the plan beyond the usual well-patient visits or major medical expenses including dental, optical, mental health care and physical therapy?

There are several factors to take into account when choosing a HMO or a PPO. HMOs are significantly less expensive and limit your out-of-pocket expenses. PPOs give you more autonomy in making healthcare decisions. Also, if you have established a good relationship with your Primary Care Physician and he or she is not covered by the HMO, you may want to choose a PPO

The Resources

Visit the following Websites for more information on health care insurance:

Insurance.com, *www.insurance.com*

Health Insurance Information, *www.healthinsurance.info*

Agency for Healthcare Research and Quality, *www.ahrq.gov*

Yahoo Small Business, *www.smallbusiness.yahoo.com*

Health Families, *www.health.families.com*

American Association of Retired People, *www.aarphealthcare.com*

Several books can be very helpful in explaining health care insurance such as:

The New Health Insurance Solution: How to Get Cheaper, Better Coverage Without a Traditional Employer Plan (Wiley, 2007)

Health Insurance (Made E-Z) (Made E-Z Products, 2001)

Making Them Pay: How to Get the Most from Health Insurance and Managed Care (St. Martin's Griffin, 2001)

Health Insurance Resources: A Guide for People with Chronic Disease and Disability (Demos Medical Publishing, 2006)

Beyond Managed Care: How Consumers and Technology are Changing the Future of Health Care (Jossey-Bass, 2000)

The Insurance Maze: How You Can Save Money on Insurance and Still Get the Coverage You Need (Kaplan Business, 2006)

34

Understanding Coding for Insurance and How It Has Changed and Will Affect Your Bill

The Challenge

Handling medical insurance is one of the most important aspects of your physician, health care or hospital program. This insurance is complicated enough that it takes special training and represents a specialization in healthcare. The most important aspect of handling medical insurance inside the medical office is to use insurance coding. These codes indicate the type of diagnostic procedure, treatment or medications being used for treating your condition and will be analyzed by your insurance company to determine whether an insurance claim will be honored and to what extent your bill will be paid by your medical insurance. The codes will be used to create an Explanation of Benefits that will be sent to you to understand how your billing is being handled. It is vital that your medical office properly prepare any coding for your condition. Failure to do so can result in unacceptable delays in receiving reimbursement for your medical treatments, or in the worst care scenario, can result in non-payment of the services delivered to you. The challenge is to understand the insurance coding process, who is responsible for handling the coding, what the record is of your medical facility in properly completing the coding and knowing what your options are in dealing with insurance claims that are not completed as needed. This will not require you to become an expert in the complicated field of insurance coding but to understand in a general way what is being done for you and the processing of your bill.

The Facts

There is a top five list of facilities that use medical coders.

- Hospitals;
- physician group practices;
- homes;
- long-term care facilities and
- outpatient clinics.

Each facility has their own rules and guidelines regarding what has to be done for medical coding and other office procedures.

Insurance coding is being seen as a growth profession, especially as the United States population ages. According to the United States Bureau of Labor Statistics, insurance code employment is expected to grow much faster than the average profession. Job prospects in the future should be very good and technicians with a proven strong background in medical coding will be in particular high demand.

Unlike physicians, nurses, technicians and front office staff, insurance coding is one of the very few medical professions where there is little or no contact with the patient. If there is a dispute or question over insurance coding, these are usually filtered through a front office staff member.

Every time a patient receives any type of health care procedure, a record is maintained of the observations, medical or surgical interventions and the outcome of any treatments. This record will include physician information as well as information provided by the patient concerning symptoms and medical history. The record will also include the results of examinations, reports on scanning, x-rays and laboratory tests, diagnoses and treatment plans. This information is organized and evaluated by medical information technicians to make sure the records are complete and accurate. The technician will communicate with the physician regarding whether the information received is complete enough to undergo medical coding.

Medical insurance coders are specialists within the medical office. Depending on the records they receive from the physician, the coder will assign a code to each diagnosis and procedure. The codes are based on classification handbooks and also are based on the knowledge, experience and judgment of the medical coder. Medical coders will then use a computer to assign the patient to one of several hundred diagnosis related groups or DRGs. The DRG determines the amount for which the hospital or medical office will be reimbursed if the patient is covered by private insurance or Medicare. In addition to DRG programs, medical coders will also use other coding systems, including those geared toward ambulatory settings or long term care.

The growth in medicine has resulted in an equal growth for coding technicians. There were almost 160,000 medical staffing positions in 2004 alone and the growth has maintained over the last few years. About two out of five of these positions were in hospitals with the rest in physician offices, nursing care centers, outpatient care facilities and home health care services. Some health information technicians are employed by medical insurance companies. Public health departments also use some technicians to assemble meaningful data.

The Solutions

Your insurance coder in the office does not simply learn on the job. Good insurance coders should have completed at least an associate's degree in medical practices and insurance coding. Courses usually required to complete this degree include anatomy, physiology, medical terminology, computer science and statistics.

As in other areas of medical practices, computers are highly used by medical coders. Software in medical coding allow coders to tabulate and analyze medical data to improve patient care, control costs, use in research services, or used to provide documentation for legal disputes over a medical bill. Understanding coding takes work. For example, cancer registrars maintain records of the facility, review patient records and pathology repots and assign codes for the diagnosis and treatment of different cancers. Registrars will conduct annual follow-ups on all patient in the registry to track their treatment, survival and recovery. This information is then used to calculate survivor rates and success rates of various types of treatment. This information may also be used by public health officials to determine the overall impact of treatment and patient outcomes for cancer and other diseases.

You must understand that the scope of duties for a medical coder may vary with the size of the facility where they work. In larger facilities, medical coders might specialize in one specific type of condition. They might supervise the activities of other medical coders. In smaller medical offices, a coder may handle all the diagnoses and treatments being used in the facility.

Not all medical coders are created equally. Most coders have to receive an associates degree with training in various aspects of medicine. Some are promoted from within a medical staff, typically after three to four years of satisfactory performance in a related position. Most medical employers prefer to use Registered Health Information Technologists, RHITs, who will have to pass a written examination offered by the American Health Information Management. Association. A medical coder should only take the exam after passing an accredited program. Those trained on the job are not eligible to take this examination.

Medical coding is basically an alpha-numeric system that is used across the healthcare system from physician offices and hospitals to insurance companies, federal agencies and international organizations. The codes are used not only for billing purposes but also to track patterns of disease and the costs of health care. Good medical coders need patience and an ability to focus on detail since a coding error can cause delayed payment of services as well as frustration for health care provider and patient. Coders are like investigators who search through records to determine what needs to be coded and how.

The Resources

Visit the following Websites for more information on medical insurance coding:

United States Bureau of Labor Statistics, *www.bls.gov*

Allied Health Schools, *www.alliedhealthschools.com*

Inside Insurance, *www.inside-insurance.com*

Medical Coding Training, *www.medical-training.info*

Insurance Coding, *www.banner.edu*

Health Care Careers, *www.health-care-careers.org*

Medical Billing and Coding, *www.medicalbillingandcoding.net*

Several books can be very helpful in learning about medical insurance coding such as:

Medical Insurance Coding Workbook 2007-2008 (Career Education, 2007)

Medical Insurance Billing and Coding: An Essentials Worktext (Saunders, 2002)

Coding Notes: Medical Insurance Pocket Guide (F.A. Davis Company, 2006)

Independent Medical Coding: The Comprehensive Guidebook for Career Success As a Medical Coder (Rayve Productions, Inc., 1998)

Medical Insurance: A Guide to Coding and Reimbursement (McGraw-Hill Science/ Engineering/Math, 2004)

Understanding Health Insurance: A Guide to Professional Billing (Delmar Thompson Learning, 2001)

35

Dealing With Insurance Disputes

The Challenge

No matter how well you believe you understand your health insurance plan, trust the information you have been provided, or have learned by experiences you have had with your carrier, you may still find yourself embroiled in a dispute over an insurance claim. Not only will you have to deal with understanding the dispute, you may have to deal with a large bureaucracy at your insurance company and through your physician, clinic or other health care providers. Dealing with insurance disputes can be challenging and, at times, frustrating, but you can reduce these frustrations. The challenge is to thoroughly understand what your carrier is offering, using good communication skills, maintaining a thorough paper trail to document what you have done and working with your health care provider, who obviously wants to get paid either from the carrier or from you. Do not give up on insurance disputes. Be prepared to do the work necessary to resolve the issue. These efforts can keep your health care provider happy, avoid problems that may appear on your credit record and provide you with some peace of mind.

The Facts

Filing a health insurance claim is a process that starts when you make the initial visit to your physician or health care provider and give the office person your insurance card to copy. Your insurance card will carry information on what your co-payment will be on a well patient visit or normal examination. This amount will be paid by you at the appointment and usually will range from $10 to $30 per visit. If there are medical procedures beyond a co-pay, the information on what is being charged to you will be sent to your insurance company for an evaluation of the bill. Your insurance company, based on your particular type of plan, will determine what they will pay, how much and what your responsibility is. This information, called an Explanation of Benefits, or EOB, will be sent to you and to your health care provider. You can then review the EOB to see if it follows what you believe are the rules of the plan. The health care provider will use it to prepare an invoice to send to you to pay for any services not covered by your health care insurance plan. The process from treatment to final invoice can take several weeks.

Most of your questions regarding your health care insurance will be answered in what are known as the policy documents or insurance handbook. This document will spell out what will be paid, what portion you can expect to owe and how you need to proceed to settle any dispute. It is usually a good idea to review this policy document soon after you receive it and contact your health care insurance provider with any questions regarding it.

Many people give up after going through the initial dispute process with the health care provider and insurance company and will just pay the amount requested to resolve the issue. Do not give up until you believe you have exhausted every avenue to resolve the dispute, or feel comfortable with what action will be taken. You may also be able to contact your state's department of insurance or attorney general to file an appeal. Check online with your state government to see how they help resolve disputes, each state's procedures are a little different.

There are several main types of aspects of your health care insurance that often arise during disputes over your bill. The information on these prevalent practices are noted and accessible by your state department of insurance or attorney general's office.

- A limitation for coverage of any pre-existing condition that was discovered prior to acquiring the insurance plan;
- pre-authorization clauses that force the patient to get the procedure approved before it is done, sometimes misapplied when the condition to be treated is an emergency and
- claims for stress-related diseases, usually caused by an accident;

The regulatory structure in the United State for insurance includes state regulations and federal regulations. State regulations can vary widely. Federal regulations may be included as part of general consumer protection or as part of Medicare or Medicaid payments.

The Solutions

If you have to contact your health care provider or health insurance carrier, there is a first tool you should have at your fingertips. This would be your health plan card, usually a small document that is meant to fit in your wallet or in your pocket. Your health insurance card will carry the name of your health care insurance provider, the group number you belong to and your personal number. It will also have a contact phone number and Website for your health insurance carrier. All of this information may be requested when you call regarding a claim and having the information readily available when you call will help expedite handling of your dispute.

Keep careful track of all of your paperwork and use it when you have to call your health care insurance plan or health care provider to deal with any charges you would dispute. Here are the basic items you should have handy when you make your calls:

- The policy documents from your health care provider clearly describing what is covered by your insurance plan and what is not;

- all correspondence you have received from your health care insurance and health care provider regarding your disputed bill and
- copies of all of your physician or health care provider bills.

To settle an insurance dispute, be prepared to have to call your insurance company, although sometimes you can register a complaint through your provider's Website. You will talk to you an insurance claims adjustor and will need to explain why you believe the EOB is in error. Always note down the name of the person you speak to and what date and time you have done so. Be sure to get a clear answer on how your dispute will be resolved and, if necessary, ask for a letter explaining these actions. Find out when your claim dispute will be resolved and be sure to call your heath care insurance carrier on that date if your claim has not been satisfactorily resolved.

Your problems can escalate if you do not take concrete action to solve a dispute with your health care bill. The bill may be turned over to a third party collection agency that will not be as interested in helping you than collecting the bill. The non-payment of the bill may end up on your permanent credit record, which can affect you applying for credit, acquiring an apartment or even seeking a job. Some consumer advocate groups believe strongly that physicians should not turn over bills to a collection agency and you can strongly express your displeasure over your physician taking this action, also vowing not to use them again. Unfortunately, the practice is still going on.

There are several common sense things to keep in mind when you are dealing with insurance disputes.

- Know your plan and be prepared to intelligently discuss it.
- Call your insurance company early in the day and avoid calling on a Monday or Friday.
- Speak slowly, calmly and politely to your insurance company representative.
- Talk to your health carrier about your claim and communicate their finding to your insurance carrier.
- Do not be put off by a representative telling you your claim is not covered. You may know the policy will be upgraded and your representative may not have that information yet.
- Be persistent and do not simply accept that something that used to be covered no longer is covered.
- Keep your cool and avoid yelling or lecturing a representative on what he or she is doing wrong.

The Resources

Visit the following Websites for more information on resolving medical insurance disputes:

Ehow, *www.ehow.com*

Medicare, *www.medicare.gov*

Bankrate, *www.bankrate.com*

Health Insurance, *www.healthinsurance.about.com*

North Dakota Government, *www.nd.gove/ndins/consumer*

State Insurance Department Sites, *www.naic.org*

Insure, *www.insure.com*

Several books can be very helpful in resolving medical insurance disputes such as:

Dictionary of Health Insurance and Managed Care (Springer Publishing Company, 2006)

The Best Healthcare for Less: Save Money on Chronic Medical Conditions and Prescription Drugs (Wiley, 2003)

Handbook on Insurance Coverage Disputes (Aspen Publishers, 2006)

The Secrets of Medical Decision Making: How to Avoid Becoming a Victim of the Health Care Machine (Loving Healing Press, 2005)

Medical Ethics Today: the Bma's Handbook of Ethics and Law (Blackwell Publishing, 2003)

Business Income Insurance Disputes (Aspen Publishers, 2006)

Section Six:

Advances in Dentistry

36

How Oral Health Can Affect General Health

The Challenge

You may pay attention to the medical needs of your body and visit your doctor on a regular basis, but you may be ignoring one of the most important aspects of your health: your oral health. This includes care of your teeth and gums and maxofacial structures. Minding oral health is not just for cosmetics. Paying attention to your oral health can have a profound effect on your general health. A good dentist can help you maintain your oral health and recommend specialists, such as periodontists or oral surgeons, as needed. Modern dental techniques make almost all procedures relatively comfortable. Both your dentist and your primary care physician can help you maintain your oral health and understand the importance of this to for good health practices.

The Facts

Many people would gladly go into combat rather than visit a dentist. They equate the dentist with pain and most do not like the idea of having someone poke around in their mouths. They will allow their teeth and gums to deteriorate before they take the step of visiting a dentist.

Recent studies have shown associations between poor oral health and coronary heart disease (CHD). The incidence of CHD has strong connections to number of healthy teeth in the mouth and extent of any periodontal disease. Diet was shown to be only a small mediator in this association.

There are other significant physical conditions besides CHD that can be caused by poor oral health.

- Chronic obesity;
- diabetes and
- caries, or an infectious tooth decay that can lead to pain, tooth loss and even death.

The figures on the links between maintaining oral health and its effect on general health concerns are compelling in the behavior patterns of visiting a dentist.

- 72 percent of adults visited the dentist within the past year for any reason.
- 69 percent of adults had their teeth cleaned by a dentist or oral hygienist within the past year.
- 31 percent of adults have lost one to five teeth due to dental decay or gum disease.
- 14 percent of adults needed to see a dentist during the year but did not do so because of the costs.
- More than one third of adults do not have any form of dental insurance.

Oral diseases are the most common of chronic diseases and constitute important health problems. They have a broad impact on individuals and society. Treating advanced oral disease can be much more expensive than well visits and regular check-ups. In some countries, oral diseases are the fourth most expensive aspect of health treatment.

Poor oral health can affect how you grow, enjoy life, look, speak, chew, taste food and socialize as well as impact your sense of social well being.

Oral health and general health concerns are equally important for children. Oral health can cause problems in sleeping, nutrition, growth, weight gain and loss in school time. Dental visits, especially for children with oral problems based on neglect, can cause 117,000 hours of lost school time per100,000 children.

In many cases, issues of oral health affect older adults the most. Oral health can be affected by medications and treatments used by older adults for other illnesses. It does not help that dental coverage is virtually non-existent under current Medicare and Medicaid coverage.

There is a growing recognition of a strong link between poor oral health of expectant mothers and pre-term low birth weight babies. Even after a baby is born the mother can transmit decay-causing bacteria through daily care giving.

The Solutions

Modern dental techniques improve all the time. With the use of anesthetics—both local and general—and high-speed drills, the discomfort of visiting a dentist can be kept to a manageable minimum. Many patients who have avoided visiting a dentist will be pleasantly surprised at how little discomfort is now involved.

Choosing a dentist is similar to choosing a physician. Consult friends and family or your primary care physician for recommendations. Look for certain aspects of the dental practice and be prepared to make a change, if necessary.

- Is the office well organized?
- Does the dentist put you at ease and explain what will be done?
- Is the dentist using the most advanced techniques in oral health care?

Oral health must be addressed for a variety of reasons that go beyond simple cosmetics. These reasons can be assessed when determining what type of treatment to undergo.

- Pain and discomfort that can disrupt your life;
- determining what you eat based on the condition of your teeth;
- changing your speech pattern and
- affecting your general quality of life.

Understanding the numbers involved in poor oral health can help you find or visit a dentist and taking better care of your oral health.

90 percent of pre-adolescents report an impact on their general health because of poor oral health.

74 percent of 35-44 year-olds report daily performance losses based on oral health problems.

Serum levels of important diet elements such as beta carotene, folate and vitamin C were significantly lower in those with poor oral health.

To become aware of what systemic conditions can be caused by problems in oral health, one must understand the direct relationship between oral conditions and systemic conditions.

Oral Manifestation Due to Systemic Conditions

Systemic Condition	Cause	Oral Manifestation
Coagulation disorders	Anticoagulation therapy Chemotherapy Liver cirrhosis Renal disease	Increased bleeding risk
Immunosuppression	Alcoholic cirrhosis Chemotherapy Diabetes Medications (steroids, immunosuppressive agents) Organ transplant therapy	Microbial infections

Systemic Condition	Cause	Oral Manifestation
Radiation sequela	Head and neck radiation	Salivary dysfunction Mucositis Increased caries risk Dysphagia Dysguesia Difficulty with mastication (chewing) Microbial infections Impaired denture retention
Steroid therapy	Autoimmune disease Organ transplant therapy	Microbial infections Increased risk for adrenal insufficiency

Oral health does not diminish with the loss of teeth. In some cases, the care will take more effort than regular tooth care.

- Dentures or partial dentures should be thoroughly cleansed daily with a denture brush or toothbrush.
- A wash cloth should be placed in the sink prior to cleaning to prevent breakage.
- Remove dentures at night and soak them in a denture cleanser.
- If necessary use a fluoride gel and foam brush to clean remaining teeth. It is not as effective as a traditional toothbrush, but can do an adequate job of cleaning.

Adults must recognize the risk and possibility of oral cancer as part of their monitoring of oral and general health. These cancers can be hard to treat and are just as dangerous as other cancers.

Any pregnant woman should see her dentist during her pregnancy for an examination and preventive cleaning. Only a small percentage of expectant mothers reported they have done this. Moreover, a similar small percentage say they were advised by their physicians to visit the dentist during the pregnancy.

To help provide dental services to those who may not be able to afford them some states are forming safety net dental clinics. Illinois, for example has developed over 120 such clinics throughout the state. A program to augment the safety net clinics is called IFloss.

Once a subject of controversy, most communities in the United States add fluoride to their public water supply to help combat tooth decay and its effect on general health. Owners of private wells should have their water tested to determine the levels of natural fluoride and possibly add supplemental fluoride. This should be done only with the advice of a public health or water official.

The Resources

Visit the following Websites for more information on oral health:

American Dental Association, *www.ada.org*

Journal of Dental Insurance, *www.jdr.ladrjournals.org*

Critical Reviews in Oral Biology, *www.crobm.ladrjournals.org*

National Institute of Health, *www.nih.gov*

World Health Organization, *www.who.int*

Hartford Center of Geriatric Nursing, *www.nursing.upenn.edu*

Several books can be very helpful in helping you understand oral health and general health such as:

Nutrition and Oral Medicine (Humana Press, 2004)

Disease Prevention and Oral Health Promotion: Socio-Dental Sciences in Action (Blackwell Publishing Limited, 1996)

Essential Dental Public Health (Oxford University Press, 2002)

Diet and Nutrition in Oral Health (Prentice Hall, 2006)

37

Understanding New Dental Technologies (Implants, Veneers, Oral Therapy)

The Challenge

Many people avoid going to the dentist for fear of pain in a procedure or ignorance over what modern, cutting-edge dental technologies can provide. Modern dentistry provides a minimum of discomfort and help alleviate a variety of medical problems: dental pain, bad breath caused by bad teeth, difficulty in eating and self-image issues from poor dental health and unsightly appearance. The challenge is for consumers to adequately understand what modern dentistry can offer, what to discuss with their dentist, how to properly choose a dentist and what new procedures can make dramatic improvements in their dental care. Good dental and oral care is more and more being perceived as a vital part of overall health care and you must take care of your teeth, gums and other oral issues as diligently as you would any part of your overall body health.

The Facts

If you are following the latest news in dental procedures, you need to recognize what is legitimately an effective procedure and what appears to be a new and exciting procedure based on aggressive marketing and public relations by providers of dental care equipment and appliances. You can determine this by carefully doing your research including looking at non-commercial, informational Websites for what are really new procedures and what are new wrappings on an old procedure.

A major buzz in dental procedures over the last few years, and for the foreseeable future, are smile makeovers. These are often referred to as cosmetic dental procedures and do not have any impact on your dental health. Another chapter in this book is devoted to cosmetic procedures.

One of the more discussed improvements in dental procedures is the use of veneers. Veneers fall into a gray zone of dental procedures, since they undoubtedly improve the look of a smile but also help prevent teeth from dental decay. In the past, veneers had to be applied to a patient after the patient's teeth had tooth structure removed. This removal allowed the veneers to be installed and not change the shape of the front of the mouth. A new veneer treatment is called lumineers. These type of veneers can be directly applied to the teeth and are made to be the thickness of thin contact lenses. This new procedure is not as invasive as traditional veneers and, if necessary, can be reversed.

A very popular whitening procedure called Zoom has been replaced with the more advanced Zoom II. Thousands of dentists across the nation use the Zoom whitening technique. The advantages of Zoom II is that it is supposed to have less sensitivity to the teeth and work faster than the older Zoom procedure.

Lasers have revolutionized a variety of medical procedures and this is no different in the field of dentistry. For many years, lasers have been used for soft applications. This has usually involved contouring the gums for cosmetic purposes, treating mouth ulcers and for performing dental surgical procedures in an almost bloodless environment. Lasers that use Argon technology have been used in dentistry to help set certain bonding materials and for power bleaching. Since 1997, dentists have been experimenting using lasers to treat cavities. The FDA approved Er:YAG lasers for use in treating human dental cavities. Despite early promise, these lasers have also been shown to cause some damage to the tooth structure being prepared. They have also tended to cause considerable amounts of heat during the treatment, sometimes adversely affecting the tooth's nerve. Later advances in laser tools for dentistry have proven lasers used for hard tissue to be more safe and proficient cutting instruments.

Improvements in dental procedures are affecting almost every aspect of dental work. The most common areas of dentistry you will encounter that may be affected by new procedures are:

- Routine prophylaxis or cleaning done twice a year;
- diagnostics using panoramic x-rays that expose a patient to less radiation;
- comprehensive examinations that use visual and x-ray evaluation;
- cosmetic dentistry including whitening and bonding;
- orthodontics with new procedures that reduce patient discomfort, simpler treatments and lessen the time necessary for a patient to wear braces;
- natural-looking tooth colored fillings that eliminate the obvious look of a filled tooth;
- endodontics or root canal therapy that increase the comfort of what has been perceived as a painful procedure;
- crowns and bridges that use porcelain technology to match a patient's other teeth;
- enhanced gum therapy to avoid loss of teeth;
- scaling and root planning in preparing periodontal, or gum, therapy;
- periodontal techniques that include gum and bone grafting and regeneration;
- dental implants to replace diseased teeth;
- new techniques in oral surgery that allow most dentists to perform the procedure in the regular dental office,

- easing of headaches and neck pain from dental problems referred to as TMJ headaches
- false plastic and hidden metal dental appliances and
- advances in emergency dental treatment usually caused by a physical accident such as a fall or car crash.

The Solutions

As with any medical procedure, you should do your research on what a new dental procedure can or cannot provide, the degree of discomfort you may have to go through and how much you can expect to spend on the procedure. A detailed conference with your dentist will help you make your decision.

Depending on the type of new dental procedure, your health care dental insurance may not pay for it, or pay a reduced amount. Your insurance carrier may decide the new procedure is not a proven alternative to a standard procedure, that it has not been properly evaluated or tested or that it is intended for cosmetic purposes and not as an alternative to a needed medical procedure. To avoid unpleasant surprises from your dental health carrier, you should obtain descriptions of the procedure being contemplated from your dentist, along with your dentist's expectation of what the procedure will accomplish. This statement should also include a detailed accounting of the expected costs of the procedure. The insurance company should then notify you in writing as to whether they will approve the procedure, and, if so, how much they will pay for it.

You should be reluctant to be the first in line for any new dental procedure. In many cases, time and use by dentists on a variety of patients will tell whether a new procedure is effective, practical and how it will affect a patient. You might want to wait for a new procedure to be used over a period of time, evaluate the results and then decide on whether you choose to use it for your own dental needs.

Laser dentistry carries great promise in minimizing patient discomfort and getting around many patient's fear of the dental drill. In many cases, but not all, a laser will eliminate or lessen the need for local anesthesia. Even the sound of the drill is more relaxing, eliminating the grinding noise and vibration of a typical drill with more of the sound of popcorn popping. Dentists have not yet achieved a state-of-art status for dental lasers. Many dentists do not believe lasers are as precise as traditional drills, but the laser is very effective in removal of cavities in the pits and fissures of the teeth. Lasers are limited in their ability to prepare teeth for crown and bridge restorations, veneers, inlays, onlays the removal of silver fillings. Lasers cut tooth enamel more slowly and not completely eliminate the need for local anesthesia. Lasers are becoming more and more popular, but the traditional drill is still faster, more predictable and easier for the dentist to use, in many respects, than the dental laser.

The Resources

Visit the following Websites for more information on new dental technologies:

Dental Resources, *www.dental-resources.com*

Dental India, *www.dentalindia.com*

Atlanta Dentist, *www.atlantadentist.com*

American Dental Association, *www.ada.org*

Health Library, *www.healthlibrary.stanford.edu*

Colgate, *www.colgate.com*

Several books can be very helpful in explaining new dental technologies such as:

Integrated Dental Treatment Planning (Oxford University Press, 2005)

Decision Making in Dental Treatment (C.V. Mosby, 1998)

Dental Treatment Planning for the Adult Patient (W.B. Saunders, 1981)

Dental Health Education: For the Education of Individuals during Dental Treatment, School Dental Health Programs and In Public Health Programs (Lea & Febiger, 1972)

As Good As New: A Consumer's Guide to Dental Implants (The Dental Implant Center Press, 2003)

Dental Science in a New Age: A History of the National Institute of Dental Research (Iowa State Press, 1992)

38
Cosmetic Dental Surgery

The Challenge

Most dental work is done for health reasons or restoring an acceptable dental appearance. However, more and more people are opting for procedures that have nothing to do with dental health, but rather a voluntary decision to improve their dental looks. These procedures are usually done by adults and may range from simple whitening to braces to surgeries that can be complicated and expensive. The challenge is to identify what you hope to acquire from cosmetic dental procedures, what the procedure means in discomfort and time and what follow-up may be needed. Similar to opting for plastic surgery, using cosmetic dental procedures is an individual decision in cooperation with a qualified dentist. You must evaluate all the factors, including costs, before proceeding.

The Facts

Many people see using dental cosmetics as much more than just satisfying ego or obsession with looks. People who sell for a business, models, actors and others who may be constantly in the public eye may desire to have cosmetic dental work done to help them in their profession. If you believe you have to have the best smile money can buy for legitimate reasons then you may want to explore cosmetic dental surgery.

Be sure to examine your dental insurance carefully before you proceed with cosmetic dental work. Your dental insurance may cover check-ups and health-related procedures such as fillings or extractions, buy may not cover elective procedures that are not related to your oral health. In some cases, your insurance company may want detailed information on the procedure, a letter of explanation from your dentist and, perhaps, comparative estimates for the procedures.

Cosmetic dental surgery does not have to be radical. The American Dental Association (ADA) says that even the smallest changes can vastly improve the appearance of your teeth.

You may be lucky enough to have been born with a perfect smile, but the years can take their toll on the best teeth. Stains from coffee or tobacco and small chips from food or grinding teeth can contribute, over the years, to a dingy smile.

As baby boomers with the monetary resources look for ways to improve their appearance and maintain an image of youth, they are turning more and more to cosmetic dental procedures. Demand for cosmetic dental procedures has been on the rise for many years. However, no matter what your goals are in employing cosmetic dental procedures, there are some things you should stay aware of.

- These procedures can be prohibitively expensive. Tooth veneers can cost between $400 and $1,500 per tooth.
- Most cosmetic procedures are not covered by dental insurance.
- Materials used for cosmetic procedures for crowns, inlays and veneers are stronger and more durable than in the recent past, but they are not indestructible. They can crack or chip and the cement used for some procedures may weaken over time. If you are 70 years old, odds are the procedures will last longer than you, but younger people may have to face the possibility of repeating the procedure every ten to 15 years.
- You must be realistic in your expectations. Dentists who specialize in cosmetic procedures are dental enhancers. They can manipulate, shape and polish the tooth material to create truly dazzling smiles. They cannot change the shape of your mouth, the tone of your skin or your overall appearance. Cosmetic dental procedures can improve your appearance, it will not completely transform it.

One of the elements of cosmetic dental procedures is the a dentist can give you an accurate prediction of what to expect from the procedure. You are unlikely to be unpleasantly surprised after the procedure is completed. You can choose from many methods of repairing, restoring or making other changes in the appearance of your teeth.

Missing teeth can go beyond looking bad when you smile or open your mouth. Missing teeth can cause your cheeks to do what dentists call fall-in. This result can make you look old and tired. Ask your dentist how important it is to your overall oral health and appearance to have a tooth replaced.

The Solutions

There is almost no limit to the scope and ability to what can be done cosmetically to improve your smile and sense of well-being about your teeth.

- Teeth whitening will brighten your teeth through the application of special chemicals.
- Tooth bleaching uses a bleach compound to brighten teeth. The procedures are usually specific but may vary significantly in cost from one dentist to another. Bleaching can be done in the dentist's office or by you at home under a dentist's supervision. Your dentist will create a custom mouthpiece that uses a ten to 20 percent carbamide peroxide. Whitening at home may take two to three weeks or two to six visits to your dentist.

- Tooth veneers are available as composite or porcelain veneers placed over the front teeth to change the color or shape of the teeth. Each type has its strengths and weaknesses. Veneers can correct a great many dental problems. Little or no anesthesia is needed for the procedure. The dentist will take a make an impression to fit the veneer to your teeth, buff the tooth to compensate for the added thickness of the veneer and then glue the veneer to the teeth.
- Dental bonding uses a material to fill in gaps between teeth.
- Dental bridges replace several missing teeth located together.
- Enamel shaping involves modifying teeth to improve appearance by removing or contouring the tooth's outer enamel. The process is often combined with bonding and is usually quick and comfortable. The results can be seen immediately..
- Tooth contouring and reshaping make small changes in the shape of your teeth and can vastly improve a smile.
- Dentures are used when existing teeth cannot be saved. Dentures, whether partial or complete, can look radically better than your original teeth.
- Dental fillings are more than just the typical metal or composite fillings for removed tooth decay. Dental fillings can now be color matched to the rest of your teeth to enhance your smile.
- Dental crowns and caps replace the top portion of a tooth. They are effective in fighting tooth decay and make the line of your teeth more even.
- Accelerated orthodontics are becoming more popular with adults who want to straighten their teeth in a few months rather than the few years needed with traditional braces.
- Cosmetic gum surgery can eliminate a gummy or long-tooth smile.

Many dentists can use imaging procedures to allow you to view before and after images of what your teeth look like now and how they will look after the procedure. This imaging is done through advanced computer technology. Your teeth are projected on to a computer monitor and the dentist can manipulate the image to show how the procedures will change your look. Imaging may not really be necessary and worth the time and expense if you are looking to correct an obvious problem such as repairing a chipped tooth or having a space between teeth narrowed. It should be fairly obvious what effect these basic procedures will accomplish. If want imaging done prior to doing a procedure, check with your dentist to see if he or she has the technology to do this.

Carefully evaluate your expectations for a cosmetic dental procedure before proceeding with it. As part of that evaluation, ask yourself several questions.

- What will your teeth look like after the changes?
- What should you expect from the physical aspect of the procedure?
- What do you need to do to maintain the positive changes from the cosmetic dental procedures?

Many years ago tooth fillings encompassed a lot of surface area on the tooth and were obvious to observers when you smiled. Dentists today can keep filling size to a bare minimum, calling less attention to them. Combined with new, lifelike materials a tooth filling can be barely detectable.

Implants for missing teeth are much more advanced than just a few years ago. With consultation from your dentist you can use titanium to be inserted into the jawbone to anchor the tooth. Implants are most effective when only a single tooth is replaced by a lifelike crown. The look will appear to be that of a real tooth, even at a short distance.

The Resources

Visit the following Websites for more information on cosmetic dental surgery:

American Dental Association, *www.ada.org*

Simple Steps Dental, *www.simplestepsdental.com*

Academy of General Dentistry, *www.agd.org*

My Doctor, *www.mydr.com.au*

Dental Find, *www.dentalfind.com*

I Enhance, *www.ienhance.com*

Several books can be very helpful in explaining cosmetic dental procedures such as:

The Perfect Smile: The Complete Guide to Cosmetic Dentistry (Hatherleigh Press, 2002)

Atlas of Cosmetic Dentistry: A Patient's Guide (Quintessence Publishing, 2004)

Current Opinion in Cosmetic Dentistry (Current Science, 1994)

Turn Back the Clock Without Losing Time: A Complete Guide to Quick and Easy Cosmetic Rejuvenation (Three Rivers Press, 2002)

Dynamic Dentistry (Link Publishers, 2003)

The Complete Idiot's Guide to Cosmetic Surgery (Alpha, 2001)

Section Seven:

Advances in Cosmetic Surgery

39

Advances in Facial Surgery

The Challenge

For most of us, nothing is more important to our sense of well-being than presenting the best appearance possible. And, this usually starts with the appearance of the face. Even for those who are not suffering from birth deformities or marred by accident, there are a variety of facial issues that may impact self-image. These could include skin conditions, the shape of the nose, wrinkles, eye problems, even image issues that affect the look of your ears. Sometimes the facial issues can have an overall health effect that goes beyond appearance. These effects could be chewing, vision or hearing impairments that can have a long-term impact. For all of these, plastic surgeons have developed a variety of surgical and non-surgical techniques that can improve the appearance of the face and help alleviate health conditions caused by facial problems. These techniques range from the nominally invasive to those that may require more complicated surgery and even a hospital stay. The challenge is to determine what issues you have regarding your facial appearance, using a qualified and experienced plastic surgeon to help recommend treatment and having realistic expectations to what that treatment can do for you. This knowledge will help you approach facial surgery in a way that will be the least intrusive and the most productive for your specific concerns.

The Facts

Aesthetic facial plastic surgery is structural plastic surgery including changing the shape of the nose, ears, chin, cheekbones and neckline and includes rejuvenative facial plastic surgery which includes procedures that can reduce the signs of aging. Reconstructive plastic surgery corrects congenital, traumatic and post-surgical deformities as well as skin cancer reconstruction.

There are several reasons why people might seek out facial surgery. Some are more important than others, but still can drive a decision.

- Injury from an accident;
- congenital defect that affects appearance such as a cleft palate;
- difficulty in eating or breathing and

- cosmetic concerns that may lead a patient to explore surgery to improve the appearance that has no direct impact on health.

New computer technologies are enhancing plastic surgeons' ability to communicate with their patients. This new hardware and software allows the surgeon to take digital photographs of the face and then modify the image on a computer monitor to let the patient see how the procedure will affect the appearance. The patient can also use this technology to show the physician what he or she likes or does not like about the current facial features.

Patients seeking a more well-rested appearance and the reduction of the effects of aging might consider blepharoplasty. This treatment can be especially useful in treating dark circles under the eye. After detailed consultation, the plastic surgeon will make an incision that will later be hidden by the eyelashes. Excess skin and fatty tissue are then removed. Recovery times can vary and take from weeks to months.

A common form of plastic surgery on the face are brow lifts. Brow lift surgery raises naturally low or heavy brows and works by removing muscles and tissues that can cause the brow to droop. Brow lifts use an incision behind the hairline and then the surgeon removes the tissue, sometimes using an endoscope. Except for possible scarring, there are few other side effects with brow lift surgery.

Chin augmentation eliminates a weak chin and provides a patient with a more pleasing profile. Sometimes the chin augmentation is performed in conjunction with rhinoplasty, or nose surgery. Augmentation uses synthetics or biological agents to augment the bone structure. Augmentation can be done with surgery or injections. This procedure needs the patient to spend time in a surgical environment. Injectables do not usually require a surgical setting or team.

Otoplasty is sometimes called ear pinning and can correct the size or placement of a patient's ears. Otoplasty is generally performed on patients between the ages of four and 14, since most children's ears stop growing at age four. In otoplasty, a plastic surgeon makes an incision behind the ear and removes cartilage and skin to make the ears more proportional to the size and shape of the head.

The Solutions

One of the most exciting new techniques in performing plastic surgery on the face and other areas of the body is through an endoscope. Using it on the face is called an endoscope facial rejuvenation. It involves inserting the endoscope, a small camera located on the end of a wire or tube, through a small incision in the skin. Once underneath the skin, the endoscope can transmit a visual image of the underlying tissues to a monitor observed by the plastic surgeon. Endoscopes have been used for many years by orthopedic surgeons to view the inside of joints, but is relatively new for plastic surgeons. Using an endoscope on the face increases the area accessible through a small incision. This allows plastic surgeons to perform brow lifts through several tiny incisions in the scalp instead of the traditional ear-to-ear incision.

An endoscope can even be used for a complete facelift. This is especially useful for patients who are concerned about jowls and mid-face sagging rather than an unsightly skin excess. The downside to this type of facial surgery is that recovery time may be a little longer than with traditional facelifts and a patient may exhibit swelling of the face that can last several weeks.

Another exciting new development in facial plastic surgery is using the tumescent technique of liposuction. This can be used to eliminate fat in the face and other parts of the body. Tumescent liposuction is where the surgeon expands the fat and tissues with local anesthesia, adrenaline and salt water, causing blood loss to be significantly reduced. More fat can then be safely removed during one session without needing general anesthesia.

Patients considering plastic surgery might be able to avoid surgery altogether by using fruit acid peels and moisturizers that can be supplied by the physician and then used at home on a daily basis. This is especially useful in treating sun-damaged skin or by using stronger fruit acids for an in-office chemical peel. These treatments include a minimal amount of recovery time and allow patients to reapply makeup much more quickly than other techniques, although a skin peel may take some time to completely heal.

One of the most advanced new methods in treating patients who wish to minimize the appearance of wrinkles and creases in the face is to use autologous fat implants. These treatments use the patient's own fat supply and can fill out areas of the face that are scarred, showing post-traumatic defects or fat loss due to aging. The procedure can be done in an outpatient setting. The fat is liposuctioned off of a fat-rich area of the body, such as the thigh, cleaned, drained of excess fluid and then injected. There is little pain or post-treatment discomfort.

More and more patients are turning to eyelid surgery to combat the look of aging including bags and dark circles. For upper eyelid surgery, a physician now uses an incision within the natural fold of the upper eyelid, allowing excess skin and fatty tissue to be removed. Lower eyelid surgery makes an incision below the lower eyelashes. Recovery time varies by patient and extent of procedure.

One of the newer and more popular plastic surgery procedures are lip augmentations. Lip augmentation allow for a fuller, more sensuous look for the lips. Temporary lip augmentation uses collagen and fat injections, which require repeated applications. A more permanent approach is to use entirely synthetic materials, such as Gore-Tex. A patient may want to start with a temporary injection to evaluate the effect and then proceed to a more permanent augmentation. A new procedure involves an injectable calcium hydroxiapatite suspended in a polysaccharine gel.

Under most circumstances, if you are contemplating plastic surgery for any area of the face, you may want to consult a plastic surgeon who has been certified by the American Academy of Facial Plastic and Reconstruction Surgery. AAFRPS surgeons are board certified and means they have completed an approved residency, is certified by two boards, has successfully completed a two-day examination and has at least two years of clinical experience with a minimum of 100 facial plastic surgery cases.

The Resources

Visit the following Websites for more information on advances in facial plastic surgery:

Board Certified Plastic Surgeons, *www.aboardcertifiedplasticsurgeonresource.com*

American Academy of Facial Plastic and Reconstructive Surgery, *www.aafprs.org*

New Image, *www.newimage.com*

Plastic Surgery News, *www.plasticsurgery.org*

Facial Plastics, *www.facialplastics.com*

Locate Plastic Surgeons, *www.1800mysurgeon.com*

Beginning Life, *www.beginninglife.com*

Several books can be very helpful in learning about facial plastic surgery such as:

Aesthetic Surgery of the Facial Mosaic (Springer Publishing Company, 2006)

Face the Facts: The Truth About Facial Plastic Surgery Procedures That Do and Don't Work (BookSurge Publishing, 2006)

Facial, Plastic, Reconstructive and Trauma Surgery (Informa Healthcare, 2003)

The Complete Book of Cosmetic Facial Surgery: A Step-By-Step Guide to the Physical and Psychological Experience (Simon and Schuster, 1986)

Your Complete Guide to Facial Cosmetic Surgery (Addicus Books, 2004)

The Face Book: The Consumer's Guide to Facial Plastic Surgery (American Academy of Facial Plastic Surgery, 1997)

40

Advances in Breast Implants

The Challenge

A major aspect to a woman's positive self-image and feeling of looking good is through the use of breast implants and augmentation surgery. This type of surgery is designed to enlarge the size of the breasts or to improve their shape and how they fit on the rest of a woman's body. In many cases the use of surgery for breast implants or augmentation is a decision based on cosmetic concerns regarding overall appearance and the desire to stay looking young. Sometimes breast surgery can be based on reconstruction after surgery from a mastectomy or from other medical conditions that impact the shape and size of the breasts. All of this surgery has different requirements, demands on the patient and the recovery time and procedures believed necessary. The challenge is when to decide to undergo breast augmentation or breast implants, working with a plastic surgeon to determine the best method for you and then following-up properly during the post operative period. With the right type of information and ability to make non-emotional, informed decisions, breast surgery can be beneficial to your look and overall attitude about your appearance.

The Facts

There are two parts of a breast implant that will affect the overall appearance and success of the procedure. Each part, unlike the days of only using silicone-filled bags, may be made of different materials and used depending on the patient.

- The breast shell forms the outline of the breast and helps define the shape of the new breast.
- The breast filling defines the size, volume and overall appearance of the breast implant.

A surgeon does not necessarily insert a breast implant directly into the chest area. More often the surgeon will insert the implant through incisions that are hidden by the navel or under the armpit. This allows a woman to present an enhanced appearance without showing unsightly scarring.

One of the most important parts of deciding on breast implant surgery is to determine the size of the new breast desired by the patient. Choosing this size depends on several factors.

- Proportions of the patient;
- shape of the breast implant;
- desired amount of cleavage from the new breasts and
- the protrusion of the breast itself when viewed from the side.

There are several factors to keep in mind if you are considering undergoing breast augmentation surgery.

- Do you believe your breast size is too small and you want to correct and enhance your body contour?
- Do you want a reduction in breast shape or volume, especially after pregnancy?
- Do you want to balance a difference in breast size?
- Do you want to have your breasts lifted with only a minimum droop?

A breast implant may be placed beneath the breast tissue and is referred to as a sub-mammary implant. The implant may be placed beneath the existing breast and the pectoral muscles of the chest. In most cases, the plastic surgeon will place the implant in the sub-pectoral position under the pectoral muscles of the chest. The sub-mammary placement is useful for women who have more ptosis, or droop, to the breast.

Although most breast implants are requested by older women concerned about the effects of aging on the appearance of their breasts, sometimes younger women are requesting the procedure to enhance their breast size. Young women should not undergo breast augmentation until their bodies and breasts have fully developed.

The Solutions

If you are interested in receiving breast implants or augmentation surgery, the first step you should take is consulting with a qualified and certified plastic surgeon. You may want to make the effort to find a plastic surgeon with an extensive background in breast implants or augmentation surgery, although many plastic surgeons have some experience in these procedures. Your plastic surgeon should be able to explain the various risks and benefits of breast surgery including the different materials available for the shell and filling of the breast implant. The surgeon may choose from a variety of materials, based on the patient's specific needs and body issues. The idea is to tailor the materials and treatment to the patient as closely as possible.

Recovery times after breast implant surgery will vary according to the extent of the procedure and the overall health of the patient. Most patients, after undergoing outpatient surgery in a clinical environment, can return home almost immediately following the surgery. Most patients who have undergone a breast implant will wear an elastic bandage to prevent shifting while the breast implants heal. Some patients may experience some amount of pain and stiffness in the implant area for the first few days to several weeks following surgery. If the surgery has caused any swelling or bruising, this should subside shortly after the surgery, and the final results of the breast implants will appear approximately six months after the surgery. Swelling or bruising that lasts longer than this should be reported to your plastic surgeon.

Plastic surgeons should have a variety of visual aids to help you see what a breast implant will do to your appearance. This visual aid may include photographs of similar body shapes or altering your own appearance by using digital photos of the upper torso and changing them on a computer to show the effect of the surgery. This type of visual aid can be very helpful in determining a new breast size and shape.

An exciting new development in breast enhancement involves using meticulous electrocautery dissection to create the space necessary for the implant. This new technique, which is now just being pioneered by plastic surgeons, minimizes the amount of bleeding into the space and dramatically reduces the amount of discomfort for the patient after the surgery. This new technique and improvements in home post-operative instructions can now make breast augmentation virtually painless for most patients. After the surgery with this technique is completed, the plastic surgeon will place sterile paper over the incisions, but there are no need for bandages. Patients can go home wearing a normal bra. Patients at home can perform simple exercises to raise their arms over their heads and speed along the healing process. Usually patients will need just a weekend to relax and recover after the breast augmentation surgery.

You are going to want to have the most natural look to your breast augmentation possible, and, to achieve this natural look, there are a variety of materials you can choose from for the appliances that will be used for the augmentation. The most common breast implants used are saline, or salt water, filled. Silicone breast implants were discontinued many years ago, but have lately been approved to be used under certain circumstances and whether the patient fits certain parameters.

There are two types of breast implants to choose from, depending on the effect to be achieved. Anatomical implants replicate the natural look of the breast as much as possible. Round breast implants can look more natural. The anatomical implant can also shift over time and create an abnormal breast appearance. You can also chose between smooth and textured implants. Textured implants can ripple more than the smooth, and, mostly do not offer any advantages to smooth breast implants.

Some newer breast implants are called expandable. This means the breast size can be inflated after substantial healing has taken place, bringing the breast to the final size required. The expandable breast implant also allows a plastic surgeon to make adjustments to the implant easily after surgery.

Another type of common breast augmentation is mastopexy, or a breast lift. Women with loose, heavy or drooping breasts will seek breast lifts rather than implants. To correct the sagging, the plastic surgeon will remove excess skin from around the nipple and bottom of the breast and then manipulate the skin to tighten the drooping area. The nipple is raised to a higher position at the same time. Excess breast tissue can be removed from the breast for patients who believe their breasts are too big.

The Resources

Visit the following Websites for more information on advances in breast implants and augmentation:

Board Certified Plastic Surgeons, *www.aboardcertifiedplasticsurgeonresource.com*

Breast Implants 411, *www.breastimplants411.com*

Greenberg Cosmetics, *www.greenbergcosmeticssurgery.com*

E-Data, *www.edata-center.com/journals*

Dr. Hackney Surgery, *www.drhackney.net*

Cosmetic Skin, *www.cosmeticskin.com/body-breast*

U.S. Food and Drug Administration, *www.fda.gov/cdrh/breastimplants*

Several books can be very helpful in learning about advances in breast implants and augmentation such as:

Cosmetic Breast Surgery: A Complete Guide to Making the Right Decision—From A to Double D (Marlowe & Company, 2004)

Breast Implants: Everything You Need to Know (Hunter House Publishers, 2002)

The Truth About Breast Implants (John Wiley & Sons, 1994)

The Silicone Breast Implant Controversy: What Women Need to Know (Crossing Press, 1993)

Silicone Survivors: Women's Experience with Breast Implants (Temple University Press, 1998)

Information for Women About the Safety of Silicone Breast Implants (National Academy Press, 1999)

41

Understanding Non-Invasive Plastic Surgery Techniques

The Challenge

Plastic surgery, whether it is based on aesthetics or necessary reconstructive surgery following a head trauma, has always emphasized, to some people, the idea of surgery. This meant that the procedures involved the use of general anesthesia, cutting on the face, bandages, a potential hospital stay and prolonged and uncomfortable recovery. However, as in other medical procedures, plastic surgeons are now turning more to non-invasive plastic surgery techniques. These techniques not only provide needed plastic surgery with a minimum of discomfort and recovery, they are also hoped to encourage people to explore what plastic surgery can do for them. The challenge is to understand the differences between invasive and non-invasive plastic surgery procedures, what is commonly being used, what your plastic surgeon can offer with non-invasive procedures and how this will affect your general health. By close consultation with a qualified plastic surgeon using the latest in non-invasive techniques, you can undergo most plastic surgery and avoid the scalpel and the hospital.

The Facts

Non-invasive does not always mean there is no intrusion into the body through incisions. Sometimes non-invasive techniques can mean minimally invasive. This means there may be some incisions into the body or the use of an endoscope, but does not include more drastic measures that, while effective, could mean the use of general anesthesia, hospital stay and prolonged recovery. If your plastic surgeon says he or she follows non-invasive techniques, be sure you know what your plastic surgeon considers to be truly non-invasive.

A plastic surgeon should be willing to present non-invasive techniques as an alternative treatment when appropriate. When you believe your plastic surgeon is avoiding presenting non-invasive techniques to your case you should specifically request his or her opinion and possibly see another physician for a second opinion.

One of the most common non-invasive plastic surgery techniques involves the use of botox. This type of treatment has been available for many years, but is still not always understood by the patient. Botox is actually a type of toxin that was initially isolated in contaminated meat. Botox can be used to treat cerebral palsy and other neurological conditions, but has achieved its modern fame through cosmetic use. The effects can minimize the wrinkles of aging in the face. It is most commonly injected to treat wrinkles and lines between and around the eyes and around the mouth. The botox, the results of which can be seen in days, is usually administered in the plastic surgeon's office. Some patients may get follow-up treatments within four to five months of the initial treatment. The injections are delivered with a fine needle inserted directly into the muscle. There usually is no follow-up recovery or pain involved.

Besides collagen, patients can also opt for dermal fillers using various types of natural or man-made injectable materials. Fillers have been used for quite some time to cosmetically correct imperfections in the skin with fat fillers used as long as 100 years ago. A rapidly growing type of dermal filler is hyaluronic acid fillers which have been found to be biocompatible and safe. Another type of filler is called sculptra filler.

Chemical peels have been used in dermatology and plastic surgery for many decades. The peels can be described as a light peel, medium-depth peels or deep peels. Light peels have been referred o as the lunchtime peels, since they can be administered easily in about an hour. In a chemical peel, a buffered hydroxy acid peel of differing concentrations is applied to the skin, sometimes in combination with a salicylic acid. Medium or deep peels can take several days to several months for the patient to recover. The deepest chemical peel is the phenol peel which gives the most dramatic results but also means the most complications including the possibility of facial scarring.

Another method of restoring a youthful appearance that does not involve a facelift is the use of dermabrasion treatment. Dermabrasion was first used in the 1940's and consists of using a wire brush rotating at a high speed going over the skin surface. The surface has been frozen by a local refrigerant spray. Laser resurfacing, which can be less of a discomfort, has been replacing dermabrasion in the last few years. A new treatment that is also replacing traditional dermabrasion is micro-dermabrasion. This technique replaces the rotating brush with aluminum oxide or sodium crystals, delivered to the skin under positive pressure.

With the rise in demand for cosmetic plastic surgery procedures is a commeasurement rise in plastic surgeons who are willing to offer any promise of benefits to sell a procedure. A reliable plastic surgeon will not promise miracles or changes you cannot reasonably believe to incur without considerable cost or discomfort. A reputable plastic surgeon will abstain, in many cases, from performing procedures purely for cosmetic purposes and will point out all the pros and cons of the procedure being considered.

The Solutions

You should do your homework on any type of medical procedure and this certainly includes learning more about non-invasive plastic surgery procedures. You can find a variety of Websites and other sources of information. Talk to your friends and family on what type of procedures they may have undergone, whether they were considered non-invasive and what was their experience as far as comfort and results.

You can investigate using collagen injections to treat fine lines, wrinkles and shallow scars. The collagen injections supplement the body's own supply of collagen, which can decrease as the patient ages. Collagen injections can raise the affected area, and smooth wrinkles and creases. Most patients request collagen for cosmetic purposes in the face, but collagen can also be used to smooth out scars in other areas of the body and make lips look more full. The collagen is injected with a local anesthetic to decrease any discomfort from the injections. Most patients describe little recovery pain or discomfort from collagen injections.

If you are looking for an alternative to collagen treatment to eliminate fine lines and wrinkles, you might consider using hylaform. Hylaform is also injected just under the skin and is made up of a viscoelastic gel. Hylaform is made of the naturally occurring body substance of hyaluronan found throughout the body. Over time, the body's supply of hyaloronan diminishes but can be augmented through hylaform. The treatment is essentially useful, too, to treat deep lines. Temporary side effects from hylaform include mild redness, itching, swelling and minor pain. Hylaform allows patients to maintain a youthful appearance.

Chemical peels can be very beneficial in lightening the skin and restoring a more youthful look, but there potentially severe side effects and long recovery times mean the patient should thoroughly research the procedure and review its pluses and minuses with the plastic surgeon. Chemical peels can, at least, cause skin sensitivity and those using them should be very careful about prolonged exposure to the sun.

If you are considering a collagen treatment you should discuss any history of connective tissue disorders with your plastic surgeon. This knowledge will help guide the treatment. Collagen is not a one-time-only treatment. The collagen is eventually absorbed into the body and a patient may need to repeat the treatments after a few years.

As they have in other medical procedures, lasers have revolutionized many plastic surgery procedures. A laser in plastic surgery can help the physician get under a patient's skin to perform endoscopic brow and face lifts, eliminating most of the cutting that was usually necessary to perform these procedures. Lasers can smooth out skin, remove unwanted hair and even treat unsightly and painful varicose veins. Among the most common laser procedures are skin resurfacing and reconditioning; removal of tattoos and pigmented lesions and the removal of blood vessels in the face and legs. Some lasers are called cool lasers and cause a minimum amount of discomfort, but their effects are less immediately visible. Hotter lasers produce faster results but can cause more immediate discomfort and prolong recovery times.

The Resources

Visit the following Websites for more information on non-invasive plastic surgery procedures:

Board Certified Plastic Surgeons, *www.aboardcertifiedplasticsurgeonresource.com*

American Academy of Facial Plastic and Reconstructive Surgery, *www.aafprs.org*

Perfect Yourself, *www.perfectyourself.com*

News Target, *www.newstarget.com*

IVillage, *www.ivillage.co.uk*

Cosmetic Plastic Surgery at a Glance, *www.plasticsurgery.org*

Plastic Surgery, *www.plastic.surgery.net*

Several books can be very helpful in learning about non-invasive plastic surgery procedures such as:

Blueprints Plastic Surgery: Outcomes and Beyond (Lippincott, Williams and Wilkins, 2004)

Beauty in Balance: A Common Sense Approach to Plastic Surgery & Treatments— Less Is More (MdPublish.com, 2006)

The Smart Woman's Guide t Plastic Surgery: Essential Information from a Female Plastic Surgeon (McGraw-Hill, 1999)

A Little Work: The Truth Behind Plastic Surgery's Park Avenue Facade (St. Martin's Griffin, 2005)

Cosmetic Surgery for Dummies (For Dummies, 2005)

Plastic Surgery Without the Surgery: The Miracle of Makeup Techniques (Warner Books, 2004)

Section Eight:

Follow Up Care

42

The Rise in Using Outpatient Treatments and Their Benefit

The Challenge

Many years ago most medical procedures beyond a basic examination had to be made inside a hospital or clinic and would require some type of hospital stay after the procedure. Patients were forced to make their decisions on receiving medical procedures factoring in whether they had the time and fiscal resources to undergo a hospital visit and stay during the initial time of recovery. Lately more and more medical procedures are handled with what are known as outpatient procedures. Outpatient procedures mean the patient could receive the treatment in an outpatient room of a hospital, a clinic or even the physician's office. The procedures offered a minimal amount of discomfort and virtually eliminated the need for any type of post-procedure stay. Patients were often sent home immediately and have gotten by with simple instructions, how to treat any post-procedure effects and what type of side effects should be reported to the physician. The challenge is to determine what type of procedure can safely be done under outpatient guidelines, how comfortable you feel using an outpatient setting and how well you are able to handle the home requirements of undergoing outpatient treatment. Using outpatient procedures wisely can mean less discomfort and less expenditure, but have to be done prudently for your safety and for the efficacy of the treatment.

The Facts

Because of improvements in sterile care and medical procedures, there are many times now when outpatient surgery or other procedures are recommended, although in some cases a brief hospital stay is still recommended for some procedures.

- If there is no need for general anesthesia, although sometimes, especially in oral surgery, a general anesthetic may still be needed;
- if the procedure does not involve a major incursion into the body through an incision;
- if the procedure has limited post-procedure side effects and lower recovery time;
- if the patient can lead a somewhat normal life after the procedure and
- if the patient and his or her family can handle the post-procedure needs after returning to the home environment.

As reported by UPI, a recent study of physicians and patients regarding outpatient services including patients with chronic problems will directly impact the quality of their daily lives. The study was made by the University of California Los Angeles and the Rand Corporation and is believed to be among the first to link better outpatient care with improved health outcomes among non-elderly patients. Researchers found patients whose care more closely followed prescribed treatment guidelines were more likely to maintain good health and had a better health-related quality of life. The study's full findings appear in the February, 2007, edition of the journal Health Services Research.

Not all procedures lend themselves to outpatient service and some patients do not make good candidates for outpatient surgery and other procedures. Among the most commonly used types of outpatient surgery are currently:

- Tonsillectomies;
- hernia repairs;
- gallbladder removals;
- plastic surgery procedures and
- cataract surgeries.

Besides outpatient surgery and procedures, many patients are using outpatient facilities to run certain medical tests. In the past, these tests may have had to be administered in a hospital setting, but can now safely be done on an outpatient basis with little or no lasting side effects to the patient.

Patient acceptance is critical in the success of any outpatient surgery or procedures. If the patient does not easily accept or is extremely critical of outpatient surgery, inpatient treatment may be indicated. Other complicating factors include a substantial distance from the medical facility, lack of sufficient support at home and the presence of significant comorbid illnesses. These should be considered by the insurance carrier evaluating the appropriateness of outpatient care.

The Solutions

You need to recognize the advantages and disadvantages in choosing outpatient treatment over in-hospital stays. These advantages and disadvantages should be thoroughly reviewed with your physician before you make your informed choice. The most obvious advantages of undergoing outpatient surgery are:

- Lower costs than those incurred with a hospital stay;
- less disorientation in having to return home;
- avoiding the distractions of the hospital stay to your recovery and
- staying away from an environment that can offer certain types of infections that can complicate your recovery.

The most obvious disadvantages to undergoing outpatient surgery or procedures are:

- Lack of access to medical specialists and support staff including anesthesiologists and nurses;

- a tendency to rush home after the procedure;
- misunderstanding instructions on outpatient post-procedure care;
- not having the support services of a hospital conveniently located in case of an emergency during the procedure or unexpected complications and
- not following through on home care procedures to help the healing process and more easily return the patient to a normal life.

A high-touch or high-tech approach to outpatient post-treatment procedures in the home involves using visiting nurses or nurse practitioners or using radio monitoring technology. A visiting nurse, technician or nurse practitioner coming to the home for the first few days of home care following an outpatient procedure can help the patient maintain their care regimen and expedite the return to a normal life. This can be especially beneficial for an elderly patient. Home monitoring, especially heart monitoring, that transmits a signal to a health care facility or physician's office can allow the physician to monitor the patient's condition and be alerted to any problems the patient might be experiencing. In most cases, these types of monitors are non-invasive and may only require leads to be applied to the exterior of the body.

Just as you would with a physician visit, you should have somebody present during the outpatient procedure or surgery, even if that person is not actually in the treatment room. The person with you can probably better understand what is being told to you regarding post-procedure care and follow-up and will be responsible for making sure you follow the physician's instructions. Even though most physicians and medical care outpatient facilities will be diligent in giving you written instructions, somebody with you can make notes and ask questions that will help you later in your recovery. Be sure to listen to this person and rely on their interpretation of the physician's advice.

Outpatient surgeries and procedures can be performed in a variety of settings including ambulatory care centers either located within a hospital setting or as a freestanding satellite facility that is either independent or part of the local hospital. Some procedures may actually be performed in the physician's office under the proper support care.

Outpatient surgery for elderly patients needs to be evaluated more closely than that for younger patients. Age does affect the body's reaction to certain anesthetic drugs and short-acting drugs often take a longer time to be excreted by the body. Elderly patients may also have other underlying medical conditions that could make outpatient treatment riskier. An elderly patient needs to undergo a thorough examination prior to outpatient surgery and relay all of their symptoms or other conditions clearly to the physician.

The Resources

Visit the following Websites for more information on outpatient surgeries and other outpatient procedures:

Science Daily, *www.sciencedaily.com*

Health System Virginia, *www.healthsystem.virginia.edu*

Medscape, *www.medscape.com*

Healthcare Cost Estimator, *www.bsbsnc.com*

Homepage, *www.homepage3.nifty.com*

University of Michigan, *www.med.umich.edu*

National Park Medical Center, *www.nationalparkmedical.com*

Several books can be very helpful in learning about outpatient surgeries and procedures such as:

American Medical Association Guide to Talking to Your Doctor (Wiley, 2001)

American Medical Association Complete Guide to Your Children's Health (Random House, 1998)

Office-Based Infertility Practice: Practice and Procedures (Springer, 2002)

The Secrets of Medical Decision Making: How to Avoid Becoming a Victim of the Health Care Machine (Loving Healing Press, 2005)

American Medical Association Guide to Home Caregiving (Wiley, 2001)

The American Holistic Medical Association Guide to Holistic Health: Healing Therapies for Optimal Wellness (Wiley, 2001)

43

Understanding Physician Directions

The Challenge

One of the most important parts of any type of medical treatment is receiving and understanding physician directions. Often times we receive these directions when we are least likely to understand and retain them. This is because we are concerned about our medical conditions and are likely to focus on only certain elements of what we are hearing. We ignore all of the directions or misunderstand what the directions and recommendations we are hearing. Not completely understanding and buying into the directions of our physicians may lead to our condition being exacerbated and not relieved. We may be tempted to brush past things we do not want to hear, which is a perfectly normal way to respond to dealing with medical conditions. The challenge is to enter into a physician relationship where we can fully understand and accept what we are being told, go through the effort during physician visits to understand and retain the information we are receiving and where we can go to further clarify the instructions we are receiving. With the right preparation and approach to the physician communication process and knowing how to deal with physician instructions, we can more easily deal with our conditions and choose treatments that are best for us.

The Facts

There are several important areas you will receive physician directions when you confer with your physician as part of an examination or consultation.

- The nature of your condition;
- the reason you may have developed this condition based on lifestyle, disease or congenital illnesses;
- the background to your condition and who else might be affected by it;
- the treatment options available to you;
- your recommendations for immediate actions;
- drug prescriptions, their regimen and the potential side effects from the drugs;
- chances of recovery;
- long-term effects from dealing with the condition and
- what follow-up treatments or diagnoses might be needed to further deal with your condition.

One of the terms you may hear as you work to understand your physician's instructions is called health literacy. This term is similar to general literacy but has nothing to do with your ability to read or write. Rather it is a term to describe understanding the nature of what you are being told by your physician and being able to act on the directions. Your level of health literacy is vital in dealing successfully with your physician and treating your condition.

You are not alone if you believe you are not properly understanding physician directions. According to the Institute of Medicine, a group of experts that advisees the federal government on important medical questions, 90 million American adults, or approximately one-half the adult population of the United States, have trouble absorbing and acting on health information received from their physicians.

A patient's overall health may depend heavily on what they are being told and what they might understand from their physician. The impact of understanding directions is far-reaching, but especially important when receiving instructions on taking medications. Medications may be far less effective if the doses are not properly apportioned or spaced out correctly during the day. Some patients do not understand their dosages and time of consumption and may take twice as much as is required. This can lead to serious side effects as well as less effectiveness from the prescription. Drugs not taken precisely in the way the physician wants can mean you condition is handled less effectively and your overall health may be affected.

It may be helpful to understand physician directions by obtaining and keeping a copy of your health records. You can do so by requesting and completing an Authorization for the Release of Information. This information will also include a record of your immunizations and drug prescriptions. Even if your physician has moved or retired, he or she is required to keep archived copies of all medical records for their patients.

Often, patients do not receive adequate information or directions because of embarrassment over the nature of the condition and how it has already been dealt with. Remember, there is very little your physician has not heard and is not there to judge you. The more information you can provide and the more honest it is will ultimately help with receiving proper directions from your physician.

The Solutions

One of the best ways to understand physicians directions is to be aware of what your condition might be before you confer with your physician. This means doing your research by searching online for sources or reading up on the nature of your condition. By knowing this information in advance, you can maximize the information you are receiving.

Make sure you are uninterrupted during a conference with your physician and that your physician is taking adequate time to discuss your condition and make you aware of what is happening to your health and how your physician proposes to work with you.

Often, physicians are very busy during a normal day and may not spend enough time to make you feel comfortable with what you are being told. Make sure you are receiving the time you need.

One of the best ways to understand physician directions is to practice listening techniques similar to those you would use during a business meeting or important personal meeting.

- Concentrate carefully on what is being told to you.
- Take notes and compare them later to what you believe you have been told.
- Repeat the information back to the physician to make sure you have properly understood what has been told you.
- Ask questions and keep on asking until you are convinced you have received the information you need.

The time you have met with your physician is not the only time you can receive physician directions. If you return home and still feel unsure about what you have been told, do not hesitate to call your physician's office to clarify the instructions you have received. You may speak directly to the physician or to the physician's nurse. In either event, this is your chance to clarify any directions you may have received earlier.

Physicians can also help patients with their health literacy by following their own methods of clear communication. Both the Institute for Medicine and the American Medical Association are encouraging physicians to forget medical jargon and use clear language when discussing a medical condition and its treatment with a patient. This practice will help patients better understand the nature of their conditions and how to deal with them and save the physician from the time to further explain the condition or have to deal with adverse consequences of patients not understanding what they are being told.

To help adequately understand physician directions, it might be helpful to have a family member or friend attend a consultation. Often you will be under stress by dealing with your condition, and this is not the best time to understand what is being told you. You may filter out what you consider to be bad news. An objective ear can help you remember what is being told to you and ask questions that may not occur to you during the consultation.

You not only have the right to obtain and keep copies of your medical information, under most circumstances you have the right to access your children's medical information, if the child is considered a minor under law, unless the child has shown a clear reason why their information should not be shared. You also have the ability to obtain medical information for a parent who may not be able to properly understand physician directions. The parent has to specify in writing you have the right to obtain their information. Sometimes this process is aided if you are considered the legal guardian of an incapacitated parent.

If you are using a telephone to receive further physician directions or to clarify what you have already been told, you need to use the telephone properly.

- Take a moment to organize your thoughts and concerns before phoning your physician's office.
- Try to decide if the problem is urgent when you call.
- You should expect to not speak directly to the physician, but, unless this is an emergency, you will receive a call back.
- Keep a pad and pencil handy to write down the information you are being given.
- Call early in the morning when most of the physician staff is on duty, this is especially true for emergency calls.
- Know the information about your drugstore if you call a physician for a refill of a prescription. This will help the physician modify the dosage or times of treatment of the prescription, or even to determine if the prescription is still needed.

The Resources

Visit the following Websites for more information on understanding physician directions:

Institute of Medicine, *www.iom.educ*

American Medical Association, *www.ama-assn.org*

American Health Institute Management Association, *www.myphr.com*

Quack Watch, *www.quackwatch.org*

American Association of Retired Persons, *www.aarp.org*

Center for Information Therapy, *www.informationtherapy.org*

Citizens' Council on Healthcare, *www.cchc-mn.org*

Several books can be very helpful in learning about understanding physician directions such as:

Spiritual Mentoring: A Guide for Seeking and Giving Direction (InterVarsity Press, 1999)

American College of Physicians Home Care Guide for HIV and AIDS (American College of Physicians, 1998)

Physician's Guide to End-Of-Life Care (American College of Physicians, 2001)

The Secrets of Medical Decision Making: How to Avoid Becoming a Victim of the Health Care Machine (Loving Healing Press, 2005)

A Physician's Guide to Healthcare Management (Blackwell Publishing Limited, 2002)

Homeopathy Simplified or Domestic Practice Made Easy (Kessinger Publishing, 2004)

44

Using Prescription Drugs and Educating Yourself on Side Effects and Drug Interaction

The Challenge

One of the most important elements of treating medical conditions is the use of prescription drugs. Almost 100 years ago prescription drugs were crude methods of treatment. Physicians had limited options to choose from in treating pain and infection. Prior to the development of penicillin, there were no real antibiotics. Often, patients would self medicate by going to a pharmacy or apothecary and purchasing drugs over the counter that would be available only by prescription today, if at all. These drugs could cause more harm than good and often relied on opiates and other narcotics to help medical conditions. Sometimes the drugs did no good at all. Later in the 20th century the prescription of drugs took on more of a systemized approach. Regulatory agencies such as the Food and Drug Administration, FDA, extensively tested new drugs prior to their being made available to the public through the prescription of a physician. Drug companies put more effort into educating physicians on the use of their drugs and how they should be prescribed. Pharmacists became more professional, having to complete extensive college courses, passing examinations to qualify as a registered pharmacist and taking their place next to the physicians as important partners in health care. Unfortunately, no system is perfect and the same applies to the use of prescription drugs. Some drugs are found, after some use, to have dangerous side effects that were not evident during the testing period, people have inflated expectations of what a prescription drug can do and sometimes patients over medicate by mixing drugs together that can cause more problems than the original condition. The challenge is to understand how drugs are prescribed, how you can best take advantage of their care and ask the right questions regarding what you are being prescribed. Taking prescription drugs properly is a challenge you must meet to successfully treat your medical condition, and this challenge can be met with the proper preparation.

The Facts

Although specific drugs are prescribed for specific conditions, there are several broad products that treat various aspects of disease and disability.

- Pain relief based on a specific condition or as a side effect of a specific condition;
- antibiotics to treat a variety of infections;

- insulin and similar drugs for the control of diabetic conditions;
- medications to alleviate heart conditions such as blood thinners;
- prescriptions to act as a dietary supplements, especially those that might lower cholesterol level;
- drugs to help control high blood pressure and
- topical drugs to help with skin conditions and other medical conditions that do not affect the interior organs.

The manufacture and sale of prescription drugs are among the most heavily funded and potentially profitable businesses in the world. Drug companies will spend and make billions of dollars in the development of new drugs. The vast majority of drugs being researched will not reach the market and the drug companies are forced to spend a lot of money in the development of a product that may never be used. On the other hand, the development of one or more blockbuster drugs that can successfully treat a common medical condition can lead to tremendous income for the drug companies. Most drug companies act responsibly in developing and attempting to release new drugs, but there is always the possibility that a prescription drug might hit the market and then be found to have negative effects. It is your responsibility to stay on top of this news as it affects the prescriptions you are taking, and, if you believe you are using a drug that has recently been found to have negative elements, you should discuss this immediately with your physician.

Unlike the bad old days, your prescription drugs are safer than ever thanks to the oversight of the federal government. All prescription drugs have to be submitted with support documentation and test results to the FDA for their review. The FDA may decide to conduct their own tests or require a drug company to conduct more tests. Some drugs may not be approved at all. The process is painstaking and takes months to complete, which is a criticism about delays in getting vital prescription drugs into the hands of patients. While there are no guarantees regarding the safety and efficacy of your prescription drugs, the oversight of the FDA provides a high level of confidence in the drugs made available to the American medical consumer.

Due, in part, to the protest of American consumers regarding the high prices of prescription drugs, many patients are using generic drugs for their treatment. These generics are made available, under law, by drug companies after a prescription is available as a name-brand prescription for a certain period of time. These generics are substantially less expensive than name-brand pharmaceuticals, while still providing the same level of treatment. The use of generics should be thoroughly discussed with your pharmacist.

One of the recent problems in the use of prescription drugs is the use of the drugs for non-medical treatments. This type of drug abuse is especially prevalent for pain killers, sedatives or stimulants. Young people are especially susceptible to misusing prescription drugs. An addiction to prescription drugs can be as damaging as an addiction to any other substance and you should only use your prescriptions, under a physician's orders, to treat specific conditions.

The Solutions

One of the more interesting developments in the marketing and use of prescription drugs is the rising use of mass media advertising for the sale of prescription drugs. While you cannot obtain a prescription drug without the approval of your physician, you can discuss the possibility of using new prescription drugs, or drugs you were not aware of, with your physician based on the advertising you are seeing. The advertising will appear in magazines, newspapers and broadcast media, especially television and can sometimes make claims that may not apply to your specific condition. While discussing these drugs with your physician represents an educated approach to treating your condition, you should ultimately trust your physician's judgment on what these drugs can do for you and what debilitating side effects may be caused by the drugs. This is not to say a physician will not prescribe one of these drugs, but should act careful to warn you about the use of these drugs.

Educating yourself on the prescription drugs you are taking or are being proposed to you is not that difficult and there are several ways you can receive the information you need.

- Websites from the actual drug company, the FDA or consumer advocate groups;
- medical pharmacology encyclopedias, usually available through your local library;
- mass media news stories on new prescription drugs and their side effects and
- publications regarding the drug, published by the drug company and made available to you by your physician as part of prescribing the drug.

Your physician is the starting point for any treatment of your medical condition, including the use of prescription drugs to alleviate symptoms or treat the actual condition. However, another vital part of your medical team is your pharmacist. A registered pharmacist is a college-trained professional who is not just there to fill your prescription. A good pharmacist can advise you on the effects of the drugs you are taking it, be aware of any interactions your new prescriptions may have with your existing prescriptions and give you advice on what to discuss with your physician regarding your prescription.

If you are using Medicare benefits to receive your prescriptions, you should know there have been substantial changes in the use of these benefits. Medicare benefits for prescription drugs are available o matter what your income, illness or drug costs are. Private companies are now setting up their own plans for the use of prescription drugs and choosing this plan can be changed every year between November 15 and December 31. Prescription costs under Medicare will vary depending on which plan you use and whether you get help paying your Medicare Part D costs. Most Part D drug plans charge a monthly premium of $27.35, a $265 deductible and a small co-payment for each drug. If you do not qualify for extra help you will encounter a coverage gap that means once you and your plan have spent a certain amount for your covered drugs, up to $2.4000, you will pay your monthly premium and all of your out-of-pocket expenses. If you have a prescription drug coverage under a private insurance plan you can drop this provision and use Medicare.

The Resources

Visit the following Websites for more information on the use of prescription drugs:

United States Food and Drug Administration, *www.fda.gov*

Medicare, *www.medicare.gov*

American Association of Retired Persons, *www.aarp.org*

Family Doctor, *www.familydoctor.org*

National Institute on Drug Abuse, *www.nida.nih.gov*

Rx List, *www.rxlist.com*

Drug Information Online, *www.drugs.com*

Several books can be very helpful in learning about using prescription drugs such as:

Complete Guide to Prescription and Nonprescription Drugs 2006 (Perigree Trade, 2005)

The Complete Idiot's Guide to Prescription Drugs (Alpha, 2006)

When Painkillers Become Dangerous: What Everyone Needs to Know About OxyContin and Other Prescription Drugs (Hazelden, 2004)

The Best Healthcare for Less: Save Money on Chronic Medical Conditions and Prescription Drugs (Wiley, 2003)

Prescription Benefits: A Consumer's Guide to Free and Discount Prescription Drugs (Benefits Publication, 2002)

Prescription Drugs Under Medicare: The Legacy of the Task Force on Prescription Drugs (Haworth Press, 2001)

45

Using Physical Therapy

The Challenge

In almost all cases, you will not be able to simply leave a medical care facility and resume your normal life. This is especially true when you are dealing with conditions that have impacted your mobility and ability to deal with pain. These conditions most frequently affect your spinal column and back, shoulders and knees. You may expect to use a physical therapist as part of your medical team. A good physical therapist can help you regain a certain amount of activity and, in some cases, may be able to help you return to what was a normal lifestyle for you, even including playing competitive sports. The therapist understands the relationship between your musculature and bone construction and can devise exercises to help with your specific conditions or aftermath of other, more invasive, treatments. A good physical therapist is a trained and licensed professional within your medical team and should work closely with your attending physicians to help you regain normal activity. Physical therapists are not just used to dealing with injuries to the body, but can also be helpful in dealing with the effects, both physical and mental, of long-term diseases. The challenge is to understand the role of the physical therapist in your recovery, how you can develop an effective relationship with your therapist, practicing follow-up exercises as required and honestly reporting to your therapist how your condition is progressing. Honesty and education are keys to working with a therapist, and, when used properly, these professionals can be of vital assistance to you in ways you may not even imagine.

The Facts

Most physical therapists will help patients in four different types of settings.

- Hospital physical therapy departments either for outpatients or to help prepare patients to return to their home lives;
- physical therapy centers that primarily work with patients in an outpatient program;
- specialized orthopedic clinics and
- the patient's home.

Physical therapists are graduates from an accredited program who have passed a thorough licensing examination issued by the state before being considered qualified to perform physical therapy exercises. Physical therapy patients include accident victims and individuals with disabling conditions such as low-back pain, arthritis, heart disease, fractures, head injuries and cerebral palsy.

Physical therapists will often consult in their practice with a variety of medical professionals including physicians, surgeons, dentists, nurses, educators, social workers, occupational therapists, speech-language pathologists and audiologists. Physical therapists may treat a wide variety of conditions or specialize in certain medical areas such as pediatrics, geriatrics, orthopedics, sports medicine, neurology and cardio-pulmonary therapy.

The education for a physical therapist is thorough and will include basic science such as biology, chemistry and physics and then introduce specialized courses in biomechanics, neuroanatomy, human growth and development, disease manifestation, examination techniques and therapeutic procedures. Often physical therapists begin their training doing some type of volunteer work in a physical therapy environment.

Some form of physical therapy has been used in medicine for centuries with records of physical treatments and massage in China around 2500 BC. Hippocrates described massage and hydrotherapy techniques as early as 460 BC. Modern physical therapy was developed in London in the late 19th century with chartered societies of physical therapy starting to be established in the 1920's. The use of physical therapy was spurred along by treating injured veterans of both world wars as well as helping victims of the polio epidemic of the early 20th century.

Many believe physical therapy is designed only for adults experiencing a variety of chronic conditions or conditions brought on by accidents and medical treatments. But, children as young as infants can be treated by a physical therapist for a variety of concerns. An infant who is not meeting growth expectations or children suffering from sports-related injuries are especially in need of physical therapy. In a child's early years, physical therapists can help with:

- Developmental delays;
- cerebral palsy;
- traumatic brain injuries;
- muscular dystrophy;
- chromosome disorders;
- orthopedic injuries from accidents or sports;
- heart problems;
- spina bifida or spinal cord injuries;
- fetal exposure to alcohol or drugs;
- acute trauma;
- limb deficiencies;
- brachial plexus injuries and
- muscle or joint pain that go beyond normal growing pains.

The Solutions

Physical therapy depends heavily on the understanding and cooperation of the patient. The patient must see him or herself as an active participant in their care and make every effort possible to follow the physical therapist's instructions when they are on their own. This may involve simple stretching exercises, exercises designed to maintain or increase flexibility and simple walking or stair movement exercises. The key is to follow directions not only regarding the nature of the exercise, but also in the exercise duration and how often the exercise is done. The physical therapist will want to push you to help bring you back into a more normal lifestyle, but it will be your responsibility to let the therapist know if you are feeling discomfort that does not allow you to maintain the exercise and may seem counter-productive to your recovery. Physical therapy is an ever-changing process that will change over some duration of time as your body reacts to the therapy and changes over time. Hopefully, these changes will be productive and help your recovery, not hinder it.

Physical therapists begin their program of treatment by carefully examining the patient's medical history. They then test and measure the patient's range of motion, balance, coordination, posture, muscle performance, respiration and motor function. They are looking for pathological red flags that indicate the presence of a physical condition that may not react to physical therapy. They will also try to help determine the patient's ability to be independent and reintegrate into the workplace and community. Depending on the findings, physical therapists will develop programs describing the treatment strategy, purpose and the expected outcome.

Although physical therapy primarily uses employing the patient's own muscles to increase flexibility and range, therapists can also use electrical stimulation, hot packs, cold compresses and ultrasound to help relieve pain and reduce swelling. Other techniques might include traction or deep tissue massage. Therapists may help patients use assistive devices such as canes, crutches or walkers.

There are many variety of types of physical therapy used depending on the nature of the condition being treated. In general, the types below are the most commonly encountered types of physical therapy.

- Musculoskeletal therapy diagnoses, treat and use of the range of physical movement to help prevent pain
- Cardiopulmonary physical therapy treats acute conditions such as asthma, acute chest infections and trauma. Not only is the therapy designed to help with recovery from various cardiopulmonary treatments, they can also help with Chronic Obstructive Pulmonary disease, cystic fibrosis and post-myocardial infarction. Cardiopulmonary therapy may involve manipulation to clear the system or using non-invasive techniques to keep the air passages clear.
- Neurological physical therapy uses exercises to restore motor functions.
- Integumentary physical therapy involves treating conditions of the skin and related organs such as wounds and burns.

If you have very specialized needs, are not responding properly to treatment or have difficulty in going to a physical therapy center, a therapist may be able to engage your therapy in your home setting. This means the therapist will set up a time on an ongoing basis to evaluate your current condition, how you are maintaining the exercises on your own and then work with you in a private setting to adjust the therapy or show you how to get the most from the techniques being recommended. In this case, the therapist acts as a type of visiting nurse, but with a lot more leeway and authority in your treatment. If necessary, the therapist will consult with your physician if the therapy does not appear to be helping you.

The Resources

Visit the following Websites for more information on physical therapy:

United States Bureau of Labor Statistics, *www.bls.gov*

Physio BD, *www.physiobd.info*

World Confederation for Physical Therapy, *www.wcpt.org*

U.S. Physical Therapist Salary Data, *www.payscale.com*

Kids Health, *www.kidshealth.org*

Medical University of South Carolina, *www.musc.edu/cp/pt*

Spine Health, *www.spine-health.com*

Several books can be very helpful in learning about physical therapy such as:

The American Physical Therapy Association Book of Body Maintenance and Repair (Holt Paperbacks, 1999)

Physical Therapy: The Truth for Students, Clinicians and Healthcare Professionals (AuthorHouse, 2006)

Orthopedic Physical Therapy Secrets (Hanley & Belfus, 2006)

Physical Therapy for Children (Saunders, 2005)

Introduction to Physical Therapy (Mosby, 2006)

Cardiovascular and Pulmonary Physical Therapy: An Evidence-Based Approach (McGraw-Hill Medical, 2004)

46

Dealing with the Emotional Effects of Medical Treatments

The Challenge

Most of us go through the majority of our lives in relative good health. We may experience the effects of a temporary condition or one brought on by an injury, but we are not used to dealing with long-term conditions that may involve extensive medical treatments. These treatments can generate tremendous changes in the lifestyle and involve adding a new level of difficulty to your life. Suddenly you have to deal with scheduling diagnostic procedures, treatments, work to confer with your physician and, most importantly, deal with concepts of your own mortality. Now, you realize that your body is a delicate mechanism which is causing you problems you never would have expected. You must deal with the frustration and sometimes disappointments of your condition and its treatment. These emotional effects can have a tremendous impact on your medical treatment, even to the point of facilitating proper treatment of your procedure. Understanding the emotional effects can help you maintain a positive attitude to what you are going through, place you in a support environment where others are dealing with similar issues, and help your physician better treat your condition. A good physician must understand there are real emotional effects of what is happening to you and be prepared to help you through the process. The challenge is to understand the nature and commonality of emotional effects that surround your condition, recognizing what these effects might be, dealing with the effects in a positive way and evaluating your health care professionals for their attitudes in helping you through the emotional effects of your condition. You may not need another member of your team, such as a therapist, and may use self-help literature to deal with the effects. But, whatever method you use, you need to know about the emotional effects of medical treatments and how they will affect you now and in the future of your treatment.

The Facts

The emotional health of a patient can have a tremendous impact on the overall physical health and capacity to heal from disorders. Most physicians agree that a patient needs a proper mental attitude to shape their physical healing. Controlling and dealing successfully with the emotional effect of illness does not necessarily mean a patient needs to consult a mental health professional. Sometimes it involves simple actions patients can take themselves to counter the debilitating effects of emotional shock.

It is not the specific event that will determine whether something is traumatic to the patient, especially in the area of illness, but the individual's experience of the event. This means patients dealing with physical illness may have different reactions to illness because of how they experience the event. This experience is filtered through the patient's understanding of the illness, what type of treatment may be prescribed and what the short and long term effects will be of the treatment and how the patient views their overall health and experience with illness in the past.

A relatively new perception of trauma is called emotional or psychological trauma. In the recent past, trauma was considered something that was caused by illnesses or men and women dealing with combat or other accidents. Recent research has now shown that emotional trauma can result from very common occurrences including the discovery of a life-threatening illness or disabling condition. Traumatizing events must be recognized and dealt with, they can take a serious emotional toll on all involved even if the event did not cause severe physical damage.

An emotional trauma usually consists of three common elements:

- The trauma was unexpected.
- The person was unprepared for the event that triggered the trauma.
- There was virtually nothing a patient could do to prevent the trauma from occurring.

There are distinct differences between ongoing trauma and short-term stress. Traumatic stress can be distinguished from stress by examining these factors:

- How quickly the upset is triggered.
- How frequently the upset is triggered.
- How intensely threatening the source of the upset is.
- How long the upset lasts.
- How long it takes to calm down, if ever, from the triggering event.

If you become frozen in a state of active emotional intensity, you are experiencing emotional trauma, even though you may not be consciously aware of the trauma or triggering factors.

The symptoms of emotional trauma will vary from individual to individual but usually will include some combination of the following:

- Easting disorders;
- sleep disturbances;
- sexual dysfunction;
- low energy;
- chronic pain that does not relate to the specific medical condition;

- depression including crying despair and feelings of hopelessness;
- anxiety and full-blown panic attacks;
- compulsive and obsessive behaviors;
- a feeling of being out of control of one's own body;
- irritability, anger and resentment;
- emotional withdrawal and separation from normal routines and relationships;
- memory lapses;
- difficulty making decisions;
- decreased concentration and
- feelings of distraction.

The Solutions

There are several ways a patient can successfully deal with the emotional trauma of the discovery and treatment of a serious illness:

- Education including doing online research or reading about the condition from books or professional journals;
- discussing the emotional trauma with the physician who may be able to place the experience in a more positive context;
- using mental health professionals such as social workers, psychologists or psychiatrists and
- attending support group sessions that include people suffering from the same physical condition and can help the patient understand and deal with emotional trauma as part of their therapies.

Trauma actually changes the essential structure of the brain. People experiencing trauma from dealing with illnesses suffer similar structural and functional irregularities. Those structural irregularities affect the main areas of the brain:

- The cortex, the outer surface where higher thinking skills arise and includes the frontal cortex, the most evolved portion of the brain;
- the limbic system which is the center of the brain where emotions evolve and
- the brain stem or reptilian brain that controls basic survival functions.

Anyone can become traumatized. Even professionals who deal on a regular basis with emotional trauma may experience trauma themselves through vicarious or secondary trauma. Trauma should never be viewed as a sign of weakness and steps should be taken to seriously deal with the symptoms just as you will take action to deal with the symptoms of the physical illness. One person may experience emotional trauma while others do not based on these factors:

- Severity of the event;
- your personal history, which may not be well recalled;
- the larger meaning the event carries for the patient;
- coping skills the patient has used in the past and has learned how to use in the present and
- reactions and support from family, friends and your professional medical team.

Besides the usual methods of treating trauma such as talk therapy, cognitive-behavior therapy, relaxation techniques and hypnosis, there are now several interesting new methods of dealing with trauma. These include Eye Movement Desensitization and Reprogramming, Somatic Experiencing, Hakomi relaxing techniques and Integrative Body Psychotherapy.

Suffering from cancer can cause the most severe trauma. During the disease you may have to deal with emotional reactions and an obsession with the treatment. Once the treatment is over and the disease has been successfully treated, it is not uncommon to still feel trauma from the event. This trauma may include feelings about your cancer suddenly resurfacing, people around you being perceived as not understanding what you have dealt with, fear of recurrence of the cancer, worries about body image, anxiety/sadness/depression, grief and loss, guilt, uncertainty emotional numbness and spiritual distress. Not all cancer patients will experience the same traumas. Your feelings will change over time, and, in general should disappear over time and the disease is being perceived as being in check.

The Resources

Visit the following Websites for more information on the emotional effects of medical treatments:

National Cancer Society, *www.cancer.org*

Livestrong, *www.livestrong.org*

Help Guide, *www.helpguide.org/mental/emotional_psychological_trauma*

National Research Council on the Effects of Terrorism, *www.books.nap.edu*

Trauma Information Pages, *www.trauma-pages.com*

Trauma Resources, *www.traumaresources.org*

Therapist 4 Me *www.therapist4me.com/trauma*

Several books can be very helpful in learning about emotional effects of medical treatments such as:

Trauma and Addiction: Ending the Cycle of Pain Through Emotional Literacy (HCI, 2000)

Post-Trauma Stress: A Personal Guide to Reduce the Long-Term Effects and Hidden Emotional Disaster Caused by Violence and Disaster (Fisher Books, 2000)

Emotional Healing with Homeopathy: Treating the Effects of Trauma (North Atlantic Books, 2003)

Five Simple Steps to Emotional Healing: The Last Self-Help Book You Will Ever Need (Fireside, 2001)

Chronic Pain: Taking Command of Our Healing!: Understanding the Emotional Trauma Underlying Chronic Pain (New Energy Press, 1995)

Healing Trauma: Attachment, Mind, Body and Brain (W. W. Norton and Company, 2003)

47

Finding Follow-Up Resources on Medical Care

The Challenge

Conferring with your physician is not meant to be an end in itself. It is the beginning of the process where you need to maintain your education. While you certainly should rely on the advice of your physician regarding the nature of your condition and your treatment options, there are other ways to discover what is going on with you. Your physician may be helpful in leading you to these other resources. Some of which you may have to work to find yourself. They are out there waiting for you to review them, but, like many aspects of your recovery, you have to put out the effort to locate what you need. The challenge is to find reliable information, identify the sources you are researching to make sure they are valid and in some type of agreement, sharing this information with your physician and then using it to act on caring for yourself or choosing the care options you believe are most appropriate to you. By taking the time and effort to locate and assimilate good follow-up resources, you can become an even more active member of your health care team and help direct your own care. You may even feel better about the nature of your condition when you discover you are not alone in dealing with this concern and learn what else is out there to help you cure yourself or live with a long-term condition.

The Facts

You can almost always find information regarding almost any medical condition by searching the Internet through a standard search engine such as Google or Yahoo. As with other information searches you will need to evaluate the Website to make sure you are receiving valid information. In general, you can trust the information you might receive via a Website that is associated with a medical association for a specific condition or group of conditions. Websites from medical schools and universities are often very reliable. These Websites will contain a variety of information including general information on the nature of the disease, news regarding new treatments and procedures, how to locate specialists in your area that can help with your condition and feedback mechanisms to the actual Websites. Some general Websites such as WebMd might also be helpful, but you will have to do a little more work to find the information you might need on a specific condition and expect this information will not be as complete as what you will find on a general Website.

The first place to start in finding follow-up resources for your medical condition is through your physician's office, especially a specialist in your condition. Frequently your physician's office will have printed literature on your condition or be able to direct you to reputable Websites. They may be able to recommend other important resources. While you are not required to only take and use the information provided by your physician, this type of information represents a good starting point in your search for information.

As you explore online resources, do not forget the basics in finding information regarding your condition. These basics have been available in some form or other for many years, but that does not mean the information provided is not as useful. The worst that might happen is the information you are receiving through more traditional methods is dated as medical advances happen quickly, but you should be able to find the most up-to-date research available based on some simple methods of searching for it:

- Locate professional journals on line or abstracts of important articles. You might be able to find these through the professional organization for physicians who treat your condition or through the larger, more general interest publications. You do not have to subscribe to these journals, but can often locate them at your local library.
- The federal and state government may offer a variety of information regarding your medical condition. Agencies such as the National Institute for Health have a variety of information from studies they have conducted or found available through other sources. Often this information is free for you to access.
- Your local library is a vital source of information that is frequently ignored. Larger libraries will contain not only journals but books on specific medical conditions. A good reference librarian can help you locate these materials, which, even if they are not available to be checked out can be copied at the library. Be sure you are finding exactly what you need and, if necessary, ask the librarian to locate the information somewhere else and acquire it for you through Interlibrary Loan.
- Browse your local bookstores or search through Websites such as Amazon.com for the latest books you can purchase. Amazon.com may also be able to refer you to articles on your condition that can be helpful.

Not only can you get information regarding your condition in a general way, you can also receive information from your physician that is specifically about you. While you may not need to pore over your medical record, your physician can give you a summary regarding your diagnosis and treatments. This information can help guide you in making further decisions regarding treating your condition.

The Solutions

Two excellent methods of finding and using follow-up resources are attending support groups regarding your condition and using online chat rooms to share information. Not only will you receive valuable advice in what other people are doing to treat similar conditions, you will also benefit from the feeling that you are not in this alone and are dealing with similar conditions that others have successfully dealt with. These groups may meet formally on a monthly or weekly basis, frequently in the clinical setting you are most familiar with. Your physician or health care facility should have information available to you on what groups are available, when they meet and what would be the realistic expectations for attending these groups. Online chat rooms can serve the same purpose in terms of sharing information or resources, but usually lack the human touch of shared experience that can help you deal with your condition. Using a combination of both could be the most helpful to you.

The information you receive will not be worth much without discussing it with your physician. This is especially true if you are receiving information that is not being readily presented by your physician or seems to be at odds with what you are being told. Your physician is giving you the best advice available and may have very good reasons for not including some of the information you are receiving outside the physician's office or why you are being treated in a way described in your own research. Use your research as a starting point for a discussion and not for a means of confrontation. Confronting your physician may only slow down the treatments you need and can be counterproductive to the treatment of your condition.

The variety of information and resources available online are perfectly exampled by the National Cancer Institute. By visiting their Website you can find links to the American Society of Clinical Oncology, M.D. Anderson Comprehensive Cancer Center, National Comprehensive Cancer Networks, Northwestern Memorial Hospital, Association of Cancer Online Resources, National Coalition for Cancer Survivorship and Children's Oncology Group. This one-stop-shopping approach to finding resources can save you a lot of time and vet the information prior to you accessing it.

The Resources

Visit the following Websites for more information on finding follow-up medical resources:

American Library Association, *www.ala.org*

National Cancer Society, *www.cancercontrol.cancer.gov*

WebMD, *www.webmd.com*

Amazon, *www.amazon.com*

Internet Medical Resources, *www.pslgroup.com*

The Mayo Clinic, *www.mayoclinic.org*

Free Medical Journals, *www.freemedicaljournals.com*

Several books can be very helpful in learning about finding follow-up medical resources such as:

All-In-One Care Planning Resource: Medical-Surgical, Pediatric, Maternity and Psychiatry Nursing Care Plans (Mosby, 2003)

Guidebook to Managed Care and Practice Management Terminology (Haworth Press, 1998)

The Medical Record as a Forensic Resource (Jones and Bartlett Publishers, Inc., 2004)

Setting Limits Fairly: Can We Learn to share Medical Resources (Oxford University Press USA, 2002)

21st Century Medical Encyclopedia with American Government Guides to Health and Medical Resources (Progressive Management, 2007)

Scarce Medical Resources and Justice (National Catholic Bioethics Center, 1987)

Section Nine:

Palliative Care

48

The Importance of
Hospice

The Challenge

Dying is part of living, and all of us will come to the time when we have to make difficult decisions on the last part of our lives. This may be caused by illness or old age, but sooner or later we will have to decide when it is time to look at care options. Some of these will involve practical decisions on finances and property. Others will involve making judgments on what type of medical treatments we will have towards the end of life and how they will impact out overall quality of life. Our families and, sometimes, friends will help us make and implement these decisions, but ultimately we will have to face them alone. One of the ways to alleviate some of this feeling about being on our own is by using the services of hospice. Hospice can provide services and care options that will help us make this final transition. Our families will also be involved in the use of hospice. Whether this palliative care is done in the home or at a special hospice center, the challenge will be to know when it is time to use this resource, whether the decision to use hospice should be made well in advance and what to expect from the treatments and therapies involved. When used properly, hospice can provide great comfort during a time of deep emotions and practical decisions.

The Facts

In 2005, according to the National Hospice and Palliative Care Organization, over 1.2 million people used hospice. This is an increase of 150,000 from the previous year. Approximately one-third of all deaths in the United States happened under the care of hospice. Over 75 percent of hospice patients died in private residences, nursing homes or other residential facilities.

There is no best time to decide when hospice is an option for you. At any time during a life-threatening illness, it is appropriate to consider hospice as well as all other patient options. The decision whether to undergo hospice care, under law, is the decision of the patient. It is certainly understandable that you may have issues with deciding to stop aggressive steps to beat your disease, but hospice staff members are very sensitive to these concerns and will always be available in advance to discuss hospice with patients and family. The patient should feel free to discuss hospice care with the physician, clergy or friends at any time during the last stages of an illness.

Most physicians should be well aware of the option of hospice care. If your physician believes he or she needs more information they can visit the Website of the National Council of Hospice Professionals Physician Section. They can also consult with state and local medical societies, state hospice organizations or the National Hospice Helpline at 800.658.8898. You and your physician can also obtain information on hospice from the American Cancer Society, American Association of Retired People and the Social Security Administration.

Hospice is not an end to itself or an irreversible step to take during what is perceived as a life-threatening condition. If the patient's condition improves or a disease goes into remission, patients can be discharged from hospice, return to aggressive therapy to treat their condition or simply go about their daily lives. The discharged patient certainly has the option to return to hospice if the need arises and Medicare and most private medical insurance will grant additional coverage for this purpose.

If you decide to receive hospice treatment at home, be aware that there is no set or recommended number of friends and family who should help with you home care needs. A hospice team should create an individualized care plan that will address the amount of caregiving needed by the patient. Hospice staff will visit the patient regularly and should always be available to answer questions, provide support and answer caregiver questions.

Management of pain is one of the most important aspects of hospice care, and hospices recognize that emotional pain is just as debilitating as physical pain. Hospice nurses and practitioners are well versed in the most current ways to manage pain through medications and devices for pain symptom relief. This relief can include music therapy, massage and even diet counseling. The goal is to keep the patient as active and mobile as possible. Hospice has a very high rate of success in managing pain through a combination of medications, counseling and therapies.

Hospice is not free but is covered nationwide by Medicare and by Medicaid in 41 states. Most private insurance will cover some type of hospice care, but you should check with your insurance plan on what is covered. Medicare will cover all services and supplies for the hospice patient related to the specific illness. The patient may be required to pay a five percent or five dollar co-payment on medications and five percent co-payment on respite care. If you do not fall under Medicare coverage or do not carry private insurance that covers hospice, most centers will strive to provide some type of financial assistance.

The Solutions

One of the ways to specify hospice care through the end of life is to incorporate this request as part of a living will. As the name implies, a living will specifies what type of care you expect while you are still alive. One of the aspects of this living will that is growing in popularity is the request to be involved in a hospice program towards the end of life. Your family should honor this and other aspects of a living will the same as if the will was used after your passing.

There are two types of common hospice care available to the patient depending on the nature of the condition and the ability to receive help from friends or family.

- Hospice centers that may be walk-ins but are frequently centers for long-term stays. It is there that hospice professionals will help administer medications, deal with therapy techniques and deal with the ongoing psychological needs of the dying patient.
- Hospice at home. During the last part of life it is usually unnecessary for a care giver to be with the patient at all times. As the condition progresses to the end of life, and based on the perception that most people do not want to die alone, it is recommended that someone be with the patient at all times. This can become problematical for those who need to lead their own lives and hospices can help with this ongoing care by providing volunteers to assist with errands and to allow primary caregivers to take necessary breaks to attend to their own needs.

Applying for hospice is a process and is not accomplished in a hurry for many good reasons. If you apply for hospice, the program will usually begin by contacting your physician to make sure he or she is agreement that hospice care is now appropriate for you. Most hospices will have medical staff available to help make this decision in the absence of a primary care physician. You will then be asked to sign consent and insurance forms for the hospice, similar to the types of forms you would sign when receiving care at a hospital. The Hospice Election Form you sign will state you understand the care is palliative and is aimed at pain relief and control of symptoms rather than to provide a cure. It will also outline the hospice services available. If you are on Medicare, the form will indicate how your hospice benefits will affect your other Medicare coverage.

Hospice patients will be cared for by a team of physicians, nurses, social workers, other counselors, hospice-certified nursing attendants, clergy and volunteers providing assistance based on their area of expertise. Hospices will also provide medications, medical supplies, care equipment and access to appropriate hospital services. A common misunderstanding on hospice is that it hastens or postpones dying, but neither is true. Hospice provides its support presence and specialized knowledge during the dying process.

Hospice is not specifically aligned to any specific faith, even though some churches and religious groups have started hospices, often in conjunction with local hospitals. Hospice is designed to care for a wide variety of patients regardless of religious affiliations or beliefs.

The Resources

Visit the following Websites for more information on understanding the importance of hospice:

National Council of Hospice Professionals and Palliative Care, *www.nhpco.org*

Hospice Net, *www.hospicenet.org*

American Health Institute Management Association, *www.myphr.com*

Hospice Foundation, *www.hospicefoundation.org*

American Association of Retired Persons, *www.aarp.org*

Medicare, *www.medicare.gov*

Hospice Care, *www.hospicecare.com*

Several books can be very helpful in learning about the importance of hospice such as:

Final Gifts: Understanding the Special Awareness, Needs and Communications of the Dying (Bantam, 1997)

The Hospice Handbook: A Complete Guide (Little, Brown and Company, 1993)

Hospice, A Labor of Love (Chalice Press, 1999)

Hospice and Palliative Care Handbook: Quality, Compliance and Reimbursement (Mosby, 2004)

Hospice and Palliative Care: Concepts and Practice (Jones and Bartlett Publishers, Inc., 2003)

Hospice Care for Children (Oxford University Press, 2001)

49

Resources for Dealing with a Deadly Illness

The Challenge

Personally encountering a deadly illness can be devastating. The illness could be related to a biological source, a virus, a serious infection or disease caused by environmental factors. Dealing with your deadly disease presents unique challenges to your physician or other health professionals. They must determine the history and nature of your condition, recognizing the potentially lethal nature of the illness, communicating the nature and consequences of your condition to you in a competent fashion, and, finally arriving at a method of therapy that will help you with the condition. Unfortunately, in many cases, a deadly illness is not really curable, but is a condition that will be with you for the rest of your life and present a profound challenge to your life and family. In some cases, the nature of your illness may have far-reaching impacts that have nothing to do with you personally. You may have been infected as part of an outbreak of a disease. You could be a carrier of this disease and will have to regulate your behavior accordingly. Your disease could be of intense interest to medical researchers, because the disease may be not-seen-before disease or mutation of another condition. All of these factors can affect you as you go through a very emotional and stressful episode in your life. The challenge is to recognize the nature of the illness, where you might have acquired it, what the long-lasting impact will be for you, who else in your life might be affected by this disease and how you can effectively deal with it, even if the illness cannot actually be cured. As with most medical conditions, education and awareness will help you with this process and a good physician can help you effectively deal with the illness as you also become aware of who else may have acquired this illness and what its impact might be in the larger community.

The Facts

There are several large categories of illnesses that can be considered both deadly and endemic. We expect to encounter these diseases in our lives, but, an even greater threat may be from the unexpected illness picked up during travel or in certain circumstances. The usual suspects for any deadly illness can include:

- Cancers of many varieties that can affect virtually any organ in the body;

- infections, especially staph infections that can be picked up through a simple body puncture, spread quickly and represent a very real health threat;
- childhood illnesses, such as measles, mumps or chicken pox that usually have no long-lasting effects on a child, but can be dangerous for adults;
- diarrheal diseases brought on by poor sanitation;
- HIV/AIDS which kills through related infections;
- malnutrition, not usually considered a disease but can represent a deadly threat for a variety of people;
- pneumonia which kills more people in the United States than all other diseases combined;
- polio, which has been drastically reduced since the 1930's, but is still a stubborn killer and
- illnesses of the digestive tract that can cause dangerous diarrhea and resulting dehydration.

Tropical and resurgent deadly illnesses are usually associated with developing areas such as Asia and Africa and Latin America. Modern travel patterns and behaviors lend themselves very easily to transference to a variety of travelers. Over the last few years there has been a notable resurgence of deadly diseases, such as malaria, that were thought to be on the wane in these areas. This points out the hardy nature of many diseases and their ability to subside before raging back

A changing and warming climate and the natural ability to adapt to survive in what were previously seen as hostile environments means there is really no safe place on the planet where deadly disease cannot strike. Because people do not believe these diseases can strike in a modern, industrialized area, there is actually a far greater threat of infection because of the disbelief that this is possible. Bacteria and viruses are can adapt fairly simply and become a problem wherever there are new hosts.

Influenza, or flu, is often considered a troublesome disease, but it can also represent a major life threatening condition with somewhat limited treatment options. Flu is caused by a virus, which are much harder to detect and fight, since viruses are not living organisms. Flu has killed millions of people over the centuries and can be easily transmitted. The flu pandemic of the late 1910's is proportionately one of the worst public health disasters in history and struck down young men in the prime of their lives as much as it affected seniors and children. Flu strains can change and evolve and researchers must scramble almost every year to create a vaccine that may be effective. Flu shots are routinely given out during cold weather months when there is a greater likelihood of transmitting the disease. Flu can also jump from animals to humans, especially flu that affects birds and pigs.

Stress in the face of dealing with a deadly illness should certainly be expected, but this stress can exacerbate the illness. Stress can have particularly debilitating effects on the reproductive system, affect the gastrointestinal tract and create autoimmune diseases which allow your immune system to attack itself. Addison's Disease is actually caused by a lack of stress which means the body received less cortisol than needed.

The Solutions

One of the most troubling aspects of dealing with a deadly disease, especially a disease caused by a bacteria is the ability of the pathogen to adapt to antibiotics that were previously shown to be effective. The bacteria can literally build up a resistance to antibiotics, forcing physicians to use higher doses of stronger antibiotics. The danger of this practice is that the use of these super-drugs may also become ineffective over time, seriously restricting physician's ability to deal with the illness in the future or even in a larger population.

Three examples of potentially deadly illnesses that are gaining more and more attention from heath care professionals show how quickly and easily some diseases can take a grip on a population and effect lives. These examples are:

- Airport malaria represents the inadvertent transport of live mosquitoes aboard aircraft arriving from tropical regions where the disease can expect to be encountered. Someone who has been bitten by a malaria mosquito and develops the disease can be ignored for malaria since the patient has never traveled to a country where malaria would be an issue. The deadly condition can be confused with influenza.
- West Nile virus made a jump to Western countries in the 1990's and over the years since has become a real health issue. The disease is carried by mosquitoes who have been feeding on infected birds. The disease can lie dormant in these carriers over the winter months and then become active during warmer weather.
- Until recently tuberculosis was thought to have been all but eradicated, especially in Western locations. However, for reasons unknown, the disease has been making a comeback and has developed strains that are harder to treat. Tuberculosis is a highly contagious disease and the possibility of its reemergence is troubling.

One of the most problematical of the aspects of dealing with deadly, highly contagious diseases is to forcibly detain those infected from interaction with the broader community. This limited form of quarantine can be seen as insensitive, but may be necessary. One recent example is South Africa's controversial policy of detaining those with drug-resistant tuberculosis. In these cases, governments must face the dilemma of balancing treatment of the individual over concerns for the larger community.

The Resources

Visit the following Websites for more information on deadly illnesses:

Lead Discovery, *www.leaddiscovery.co.uk*

PBS, *www.pbs.org/WGBH/rxforsurvival/series/diseases*

The Guardian, *www.guardian.co.uk*

Medical Moment, *www.medicalmoment.org*

National Marrow Donor Program, *www.marrow.org*

National Cancer Institute, *www.cancer.gov*

National Institute of Child Health & Human Development, *www.nichd.nih.gov*

Several books can be very helpful in learning about deadly illnesses such as:

Deadly Emotions: Understand the Mind-Body-Spirit Connection that Can Heal or Destroy You (Thomas Nelson, 2003)

The Pathological Protein: Mad Cow, Chronic Wasting and Other Deadly Prion Diseases (Springer, 2006)

The Deadly Truth: A History of Disease in America (Harvard University Press, 2002)

The Illness Narratives: Suffering, Healing, and the Human Condition (Basic Books, 1989)

The Social Medicine Reader, Second Edition, Vol. One: Patients, Doctors, and Illness (Duke University Press, 2005)

When Chronic Illness Enters Your Life (Rest Ministries Publishers, 2002)

50
Involving Family and Friends

The Challenge

You should not face your medical condition alone. You have the resources of your family and your friends to help you. These support givers can help you acquire and understand the information you are receiving, make sure you are properly following physician instructions, and, sometimes just provide a shoulder to cry on when the implications of your condition seem to be too much to bear. Most of our family and friends want to be available to help because they care about you. They cannot act as your assistant physician but they can be an absolutely vital part of your healthcare team. The challenge is to identify what family and friends can reasonably be asked to do, finding ways to involve them, not to rely too heavily on people who have their own lives and concerns to deal with and understanding their place in your health care treatment. When allowed to enter your life, your family and friends can be instrumental in helping you deal with your condition and return to help. They can help you alter your lifestyle to avoid a recurrence of the condition. You must place their assistance into context and use what you can while always letting your family and friends know how much you value their help. Remember, you are not in this alone and no one who is close to you wants you to feel this way.

The Facts

You may not need a friend or family member's help in caregiving during a non-serious or non life-threatening medical condition. The stress of this condition may be so low is that you can handle the information and make your decisions. However, there are some types of conditions that may need the help of family and friends:

- Heart conditions;
- cancer;
- eye conditions;
- motion problems and
- psychotherapy that needs practical care.

There are a variety of services family and friends can help provide you:

- Visiting the physician to help you understand directions and ask questions;

- picking up prescriptions for you if you are home bound or do not have readily available transportation;
- lay out your prescriptions, usually using pill sorters, to make sure you are taking the proper medications at the proper time;
- shopping for medical supplies and food;
- taking your temperature and doing other non-extensive home tests;
- communicating with your physician regarding your condition
- preparing food, sometimes in advance, doing basic cleaning and helping with laundry chores;
- paying bills and assisting with finances; and
- providing psychological support for you by being available to listen to your concerns and fears and make sure you know you have someone who is willing to talk to you and listen to what you feel.

A good physician will understand the concept of family dynamics when dealing with the help of family members in dealing with their patients. They know that family can be a major factor in the recovery of their patient, but that the dynamics of the individual family will affect how they deal with the family members. A good physician will take the time to learn about the family dynamics in a non-intrusive way. They may discover the primary caregiver in the family may not be the family decision maker or accompany the patient to physician consultations. Family members may disagree about treatment options. A patient may have a different definition of family that differs from those who are related by blood. The physician may use genograms and ecomaps along with extensive meetings with the family to chart the dynamics.

The Solutions

The first place family or friends can help with your medical conditions is during the consultations and examinations you will have with your physician. Often, we are receiving vital information and being asked important questions during a time when our attention is turned inward from the shock of hearing about the condition. During this time, until we have learned how to deal with hearing about our medical condition, we may not be understanding properly what we are being told or are expected to understand. We may be asked questions or given alternatives to our treatment options that do not make sense. Your physician will probably not expect an answer from you immediately, but will need your feedback and approval for treatment in the near future. A friend or family member with good listening skills can sit in on these consultations and make notes about what you are being told. They may also be able to ask questions that would not occur to you at the time. The physician must know that this person has your approval to hear about your medical condition, and, while this person will not be the one to directly communicate a response to the physician, you will talk to them about what you are being told to process the information being given to you. It is possible you may go home or to a more relaxing environment to further discuss your consultation, removing the stress of being in a medical environment to help you make your decisions. The key is to find someone who can listen, understand what is being told to you, make clear notes on the information and then help you later decide on what you might want to do.

Remember, a family member or friend is not an educated or paid health provider. They will be there for you to help you as much as possible, but you must expect they have their own lives to lead and may not always be readily available. The answer is to let the family and friend know what you need help with and give them plenty of notice of when you will need the help. This will help facilitate the aid you are getting and avoid feelings of resentment from your family member or friend that can lead to not helping you as much as possible, and, maybe, stop helping altogether out of frustration or a feeling of being unappreciated.

Not all medical conditions will require the participation of your family or friends to help with. Many medical conditions can easily be dealt with on your own. But, depending on your condition, its progress and your age, there are some broad categories of medical conditions that can be helped by family or friends:

- Conditions caused by injury that will limit your mobility and ability to leave the house including broken bones, pulled muscles and internal injuries that will take time to heal;
- long-term, potentially fatal diseases such as cancer or HIV/AIDS where the patient may still need a visiting nurse to help with medical testing and treatments, but may require help with some daily activities that have become difficult to perform;
- mental disorders that will affect the ability to do basic functions such as mild dementia, addiction recovery or Alzheimer's disease, keeping in mind there may come a time when the patient has to enter a regular medical care facility for long-term care and
- temporary conditions that have either recently developed and being coped with by the patient or will alleviate over time and allow the patient to reintegrate into society and take care of themselves.

One benefit of using a bilingual family or friend is he or she can understand, in English, what is being told to you by your physician and then translate this information to you. While it is certainly possible to find healthcare providers who speak other languages, especially Spanish, they can be hard to locate and may not be exactly what you are looking for. The challenge of finding a multi-lingual physician in a more rural area can be even more difficult. This translation ability can be vital in treating your medical condition.

To help your family and friends honor your wishes if you become unable to make decisions, you may want to create a medical advance directive. This document will help guide the family member or friend do what you would have done. They protect your rights as a patient. Similar to the medical directive is the Medical Power of Attorney which allows you to appoint someone as your agent to make health care decisions for you if you cannot do so for yourself. An attorney can help you draw up an advanced medical directive, power of attorney or living will to facilitate the process when and if the time comes.

The Resources

Visit the following Websites for more information on the role of family and friends:

National Library of Medicine Gateway, *www.gateway.nlm.nigh.gov*

Palliative Care Victoria, *www.pallcarevic.asn.au*

My Whatever, *www.mywhatever.com*

Dementia Care Central, *www1.dementiacarecentral.com*

University Health System, *www.universityhealthsystem.com*

Nature, *www.nature.com*

Pub Med, *www.ncbi.nlm.nih.gov*

Several books can be very helpful in learning about the role of family and friends in medical care such as:

Surviving Modern Medicine: How to Get the Best from Doctors, Family, and Friends (Rutgers University Press, 1998)

Harvard Medical School Family Health Guide (Free Press, 2004)

Alzheimer's Early Stages: First Steps for Families, Friends and Care-Givers (Hunter House, 2003)

American College of Physicians Home Care Guide for HIV and AIDS: For Family and Friends Giving Care at Home (American College of Physicians, 1998)

100 Q&A About Caring for Family or Friends with Cancer (Jones and Bartlett Publishers, 2004)

Understanding Family Care: A Multi-Dimensional Model of Caring and Coping (Open University Press, 1996)

Holistic Treatments

The Challenge

Many patients are looking for what they believe are viable alternatives to traditional medical treatments of drugs and surgery. The use of massage and acupuncture have been used for many years. Now those treatments are being joined by the use of yoga, aromatherapy, group discussions and, in some cases, even crystals or other inert substances. All of these are grouped under the heading of holistic medicine or homeopathy therapies. Whether these treatment can be as physically effective as using traditional medical treatments or consulting a physician, they can often offer psychological assistance to the patient and, thus, speed along the healing process and sense of well being. The challenge is to recognize what types of holistic treatments are available, what they can do to treat specific conditions, maintain realistic expectations and use them effectively in conjunction with other medical treatments. It is doubtful if holistic treatments can ever replace the benefits of surgery, but few physicians will completely discount the use of holistic therapy. By carefully using these treatments and evaluating the qualifications and proven track records of the holistic therapist, you may be able to aid in your recovery in ways you did not consider when initially visiting your physician.

The Facts

The American Holistic Medical Association says that holistic medicine is the art and science of healing that addresses care of the whole person including the body, mind and spirit. The practice of holistic medicine marries conventional and complimentary therapies to promote optimal health and to prevent and treat disease by addressing contributing factors.

Holistic medicine sees every person as a unique individual, rather than an example of a particular disease. Disease is understood by holistic medicine as the result of physical, emotional, spiritual, social and environmental imbalance. Healing is believed to take place naturally when these aspects of life are brought into proper balance.

One of the first examples of holistic medicine that is now seen in a more respectable light is that of chiropracty or osteopathy. This older science stresses the manipulation of the spine, related bones and muscle structures to facilitate healing. Many orthopedic surgeons may now recommend chiropractic medicine for help in healing joint and muscle pain with the understanding that the patient may still need some type of medication and possibly surgery. Most physicians part company with chiropractors or osteopaths when they claim their techniques can help with illnesses and medical conditions that do not immediately impact the joints or related muscle tissues. Physicians, by and large, do not believe these claims of being able to provide cures without medication and stress the patient should seek out common medical therapies to meet specific conditions.

An ethical holistic practitioner keeps the practice in context. He or she views the patient as being ultimately responsible for his or her well being, fosters and maintains a partnership with the patient using therapies that feel comfortable and non-threatening and evaluates and recommends treatment options that address both the cause of a condition as well as the symptoms. The holistic practitioner may choose or recommend from a variety of conventional and alternative treatments and therapies. The practitioner and patient/client work together to develop a partnership that will find an optimal course of therapies. This partnership can be a powerful approach to healing and is considered the cornerstone of the holistic philosophy.

Besides the partnership and trusting relationship developed between a holistic practitioner and the patient there are other perceived benefits of holistic treatments:

- The central role of the patient's lifestyle, beliefs, observations and habits are honored. Holistic medicine strives to recognize the person who has the illness to be more important than the type of illness the patient is manifesting.
- Holistic medicine starts with treatment options that are least likely to do harm. These methods are often less costly than conventional drugs or therapies.
- Holistic medicine is part of a world view which hopes to achieve societal changes through respect for the individual patient and for the nature of diversity to an integrative model of healing. This medicine believes that healing must take place on all levels, individual, social, cultural and planetary for the survival and happiness of life on earth.

Alternative therapies are those defined as not normally offered by conventional medical personnel. They may include, but are not limited to, nutrition, herbal medicine, spinal manipulation, body work medicine, energy medicine, spiritual attunement, relaxation training and stress management, biofeedback and acupuncture.

The Solutions

The holistic practitioner does not consider him or herself to be the only instrument of attaining good health in a patient and correcting medical conditions. The practitioner is meant to be a guide, mentor and role model. The patient is expected to do the majority of the work involved in holistic healing. This work might mean changing lifestyle, finding new beliefs and forgetting old habits in order to facilitate healing. Holistic methods can range from medication to meditation and many ideas in between.

Herbal medicines and the use of dietary supplements are often heavily recommended by holistic physicians. They see these medicines as viable alternatives to prescription drugs and can provide relief from a medical condition without relying on antibiotics or standard pain killers. These drugs can be purchased through the Internet or from catalogs, or from stores specializing in the sale of herbal medicines and diet supplements. Undoubtedly some of these drugs may have a positive effect on the human body, especially if they relieve stress or help with weight loss. But, you must be aware that these drugs are available without the type of testing regular pharmaceuticals receive from the Food and Drug Administration. Their effects may be more psychological than physical and can carry side effects that are not recognized by practitioners. It is not uncommon for a non-prescription drug to be banned from sale because it has been found to be harmful. As you would with regular prescription drugs, you should ask careful questions about the drug's background and make sure you follow strict instructions in taking it.

Therapeutic massage is another therapy that has been seen in the past as being beneficial in dealing with joint or muscle conditions. These therapists have to undergo a thorough training and apprenticeship program and pass medical examinations before practicing, since massage therapy that is not properly administered can cause as much harm as good. Some holistic practitioners may advertise they are experts in massage, but you should carefully check their credentials before undergoing potentially dangerous massage therapy. If you feel the massage is causing more discomfort than it is alleviating, you may want to consult your physician or visit another massage therapist for a second opinion and schedule of treatments.

You can find holistic practitioners occasionally from your physicians. Friends, family and colleagues who have suffered similar conditions may also be able to help you find good holistic medicine. You can also find a directory of holistic practitioners in several disciplines in your area by contacting the American Holistic Medical Association at *www.holisticmedicine.org* or by calling the American Holistic Health Association at 714.779.6157.

Reputable holistic physicians will not claim they can fix your problem, only find the interaction of factors that may be contributing to your condition. Before working on you they will ask for your Informed Consent. Informed consent is the process by which a physician helps a patient arrive at an informed decision regarding treatment options. Your hopes and fears must be addressed as well as psychological factors and family expectations.

Not all medical insurance plans will cover holistic medical techniques, and, if they do, these techniques may be limited to chiropracty, massage or acupuncture. As a rule, most holistic healers are not covered under HMO type of medical insurance. As with other types of medicine, you should check with your insurance carrier before you receive the treatment to see if your treatment is covered and to what extent.

Holistic medicine is often treated skeptically by other physicians because there are no empirical tests available for holistic medicine. Thus, the efficacy of holistic therapies is widely disputed ranging from it cannot hurt to worry that holistic treatments will be relied upon more than conventional treatments. Physicians see holistic therapies as not completely safe and will needlessly delay a patient from seeking conventional therapies.

The Resources

Visit the following Websites for more information on holistic medicine treatments:

American Holistic Health Association, *www.holisticmed.com*

American Holistic Medicine Association, *www.holisticmedicine.org*

National Center for Complementary and Alternative Medicine, *www.ncaam.nih.gov*

Alternative Cancer Information, *www.altcancerinfo.org*

Natural Medicines Comprehensive Database, *naturaldatabase.com*

The British Library, *www.blu.uk/collections/business/compmein*

Chopra Center, *www.chopra.com*

Several books can be very helpful in learning about holistic medicine such as:

The Complete Self-Care Guide to Holistic Medicine: Treating Our Most Common Ailments (Tarcher, 1999)

The American Holistic Health Association Complete Guide to Alternative Medicine (Warner Books, 1997)

The Complete Book of Chinese Medicine: A Holistic Approach to Physical, Emotional and Mental Health (Cosmos Publishing, 2002)

Culpepper's Medicine: A Practice of Western Holistic Medicine (Element Books, 1997)

Child Health Guide: Holistic Pediatrics for Parents (North Atlantic Books, 2005)

Complementary and Alternative Medicine for Older Adults: Holistic Approaches to Healthy Aging (Springer Publishing Company, 2006)